TOP 3 FIX

Bob and Brad's (and Rick's)
3 Most Effective Exercises
to Solve Pain from Headaches to Plantar Fasciitis

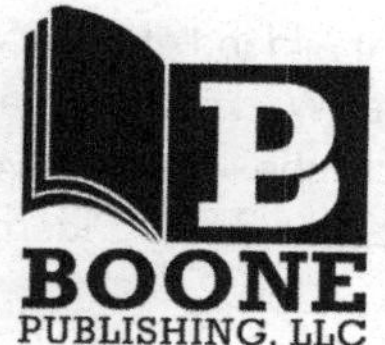

Boone Publishing, LLC

Project Editor: Noah Charney

Interior Layout & Design: Urška Charney

Medical Illustrations:
Martin Huber (mdhuber@gmail.com)
Meghan Lewis (meghan.marie.lewis@gmail.com)

Exercise Photographs: Scott Sturgis/Big-Fish Design

Boone Publishing, LLC www.BoonePublishing.com

Library of Congress Control Number: 2023949424

Library of Congress Subject Heading:

1. Backache—Physical Therapy—Treatment—Hand- books, manuals, etc. 2. Backache—Popular Works. 3. Back—Care & Hygiene—Popular Works. 4. Backache— Exercise Therapy. 5. Self-care, Health—Handbooks, manuals, etc. 6. Backache—Alternative Treatment. 7. Backache—Exercise Therapy. 8. Backache—Prevention. I. Title: Top 3 Fix. Olderman, Rick. III. Title.

ISBN 978-0-9819152-0-3

Printed in the United States of America Version 1.0
Printed in the United States of America

CONTENTS

[torn]LOGUE

There Are a Few Things You Should Know Immediately

1. Most of the exercises and habit changes that will be presented are repeated throughout the book. For example, you will see some of the same exercises for neck pain, neck hump, and headaches. That doesn't mean they won't work—in fact, the opposite. It simply means that the same root source can cause pain in multiple locations, and some fixes will sort out more than one issue. We wanted to make it easy and convenient for you to treat your particular pain. If you want to treat neck pain, for instance, we direct you to Chapter 4, and the exercises located there. There is no need to refer you to multiple portions of the book.

2. Sure, you can turn to the chapter that is relevant to you and start doing the exercises. However, if you want to know **why** we are having you do the exercises, I recommend reading Chapter 3 (How the Upper Body System Works) before reading any of chapters 4-8. Same goes for reading Chapter 9 (How the Lower Body System Works) before reading any of chapters 10-19.

3. Videos are available for all exercises and habit changes presented in this book. Go to the website **top3fix.com** and enter your email and the code TOP3FIX to access them.

4. Make sure that you are doing all the exercises and implementing habit changes. **Do not skip any of the exercises or habit changes.** They all carry equal importance. Also, make sure you do the exercises and habit changes correctly.

5. Have faith that these exercises will work. The 100+ testimonials provided in this book will let you know that they do. The testimonials are from a mix of people who have used Rick's system at his clinic, watched his videos, or read his books.

CHAPTER 1

Why Top 3 Fix and How to Use This Book

I am fairly certain of one thing. It's not your desire to curl up with a book on pain and spend an afternoon reading it.

That is exactly why we wrote this book.

It's meant for you to skip to the section that covers your issue and immediately discover the three best exercises you can do to address your problem.

The goal of the Top 3 Fix approach is to provide you with the three best exercises that treat a particular painful condition. We like to think that we provide the three silver bullets–magical solutions to a previously unsolvable problem–of treatment. We believe we have found exercises that are just that: magical.

Why three exercises? Why not four or five? This is not a new idea. I've read that the army often employs the "rule of three." Give someone three goals or tasks and they have a good chance of completing them. Increase that number to four and compliance plummets.

We find that the same is true with our patients. Give them too many exercises, and they fail to do them.

As physical therapists, we know that, for patients, the best motivation to do exercises is seeing positive results from doing them. If patients get some early "wins," they stick with their program. Therefore, we know that the exercises we prescribe must darn well be the top exercises with the best chances of working.

We have put a system in place for doing just that. With Top 3 Fix, we've attempted to find the three best exercises you can perform and the best habits you can change to treat your pain. The idea is to achieve the best overall result with the least amount of effort.

An expert is someone we inherently trust when it comes to treating a person whose issue falls within their field of study. Our system starts with our expert, Rick Olderman, MSPT, a renowned specialist in solving chronic pain. He has invariably proven himself with his body of work. We believe that Rick can give some of the best advice on the planet.

Let me describe how we developed a relationship with Rick Olderman. As a member of "Bob and Brad," and a producer of our podcast, I am continually exposed to some of the most top-notch talent in the world. So, I recognize talent when I see it.

First, I (Bob) read six of Rick's self-help books. I found his ideas to be very insightful, so I invited him to be on the Bob and Brad podcast. He was an extremely impressive guest, so I started purchasing some of his (very inexpensive) online programs. I had terrible pain in my right upper trap, which I had used several methods to treat. These other methods were modestly successful, but within a month the pain had come roaring back. Then I employed Rick's method: it decisively took the pain away, and it stayed away.

A friend, who had been a Director of Nursing,

"We believe we have found exercises that are just that. Magical!"

called me because she was having horrendous pain in both knees. She couldn't sleep at night, and she was taking various medications and using CBD cream with no effect. She was desperate. I had her try Rick's program. She began to feel relief within a few days. She is currently off all pain meds and is pain-free.

I then participated in Rick's instructional program for physical therapists. It's an in-depth program the likes of which I had never experienced. His focus is treating the root of the problem, which isn't always found where you think it would be. For example, the cause of neck pain is often a displaced shoulder blade.

I took what I had learned from Rick and began to apply it to my patients.

My wife was suffering from back pain. I had been using other treatments for her, but her back pain had progressed to the point that she was going to give up bowling. On Rick's program, her pain got better in two days, and she was bowling pain-free in a week. I was a genius in her eyes. But it was all Rick.

As a further example (I could give many more), I had Rick see my daughter, Jamie, through online telehealth. I had treated her, but I was stuck as to what to do to resolve her persistent pain and numbness in her right hand and pinky. He confidently led her down a successful treatment path.

I could go on and on with additional examples. I jokingly refer to Rick as "Jesus-like" because of his ability to cure the painful. I consider Rick to be the best physical therapist I know. He is simply amazing.

Now, we understand that patients would do better if they did more than just three exercises or stretches. But as human nature would have it, if we prescribe patients with more exercises, they may not do any at all and therefore will not improve.

Patients would also do better if treatment advice were individualized. Unfortunately, most people don't have access to top-notch physical therapy. That is why we chose the top three exercises for each condition.

Feel free to skip to the section of the book that's relevant to you and dive into the three exercises that are right for your problem. In addition, take a look at the habits you should change.

Our goal is to get you to commit to performing those three exercises. In addition, we ask that you change a few habits in your life, for your own benefit, of course. Do this, and you stand a good chance of experiencing pain relief.

How often should you do the exercises? I think sprinkling them throughout the day works best. I try to develop cues for performing the exercises, like exercising upon waking or after a meal or doing a doorway stretch every time I walk through a door. My sister (she's a teacher) does her exercises between classes (she has just two minutes, but even that is enough).

CHAPTER 2

Why You Should Read This Book

I (Bob) have been a physical therapist for 38 years. Because of the Bob and Brad channel, I've had access to some of the best doctors, athletic trainers, and physical therapists in the field. Despite that privilege, when I was exposed to Rick Olderman's work, it was like I was removing a blindfold of ignorance. He could explain things I had wondered about for years. I truly questioned why everyone in my field didn't know who Rick Olderman was.

I ended up taking Rick Olderman's full course for professionals. Since then, there are times when I feel like a miracle worker. Just two days ago, I saw an employee with back pain. I assigned him three stretches and one habit to change. He is 90% better today.

I don't know how much time I have on Earth, but I am going to spend the remainder of my days shouting from the rooftops about Rick Olderman and his methods.

I know it will be hard for many to believe that these exercises and habit changes will help them. But here's the secret: the reason many of you have not gotten better is that you have been treating the wrong area. Who would think that most neck, shoulder, or headache problems will not get better unless you treat the shoulder blades? Or that most back, hip, or sacroiliac joint issues will not get better unless you learn to use and engage your glutes?

Rick has used his vast experience in the clinical setting to narrow down his exercise choices to what he determined to be the best three. What I like most about the exercises and habit changes is that they are relatively simple to do. If you have trouble understanding them, you can watch our free videos on our Top 3 Fix website. Enter the code TOP3FIX in the code box.

I am going to use the rest of this chapter to provide real-life testimonials of the effectiveness of Rick's program. In this chapter, as well as on the back cover and spread throughout the book, **I have included over 100 testimonials.** A little much, perhaps, but it proves a point:

"More than 100 people have enthusiastically reported that the excersies prescribed by Rick changed their lives for the better."

this really works. More than 100 people have enthusiastically reported that the exercises prescribed by Rick changed their lives for the better. Although these testimonials were not written about this book, they were written in praise of the exercises presented in this book. These are from people who saw Rick in person, signed up for one of his video programs, or read one of his previous books. There are times I substituted the words "Rick's system" for the name of his former practice, "Body in Balance," as, either way, it was his system that made the person better, allowing them to cast aside their pain.

I know, I know. Including 100+ testimonials is ridiculous. I am well aware that it is overkill. But I look at it this way: experiencing relief from pain is one of the greatest gifts a person can receive.

Please note that any testimonial reference to a book is NOT referring to this book. Rather, it is a reference to a previous book by Rick Olderman. The testimonials presented here are in praise of Rick's techniques, showcased in his previous books, online videos, courses, and in person. However, this book presents the same exercises praised in the testimonials, so the praise is entirely relevant.

You can't imagine the agony, anxiety, and depression people experience due to chronic pain. These are 100+ humans whose lives were made significantly better because of the knowledge, exercises, and guidance provided by Rick Olderman. So, I decided that I don't care how many pages the testimonials add to this book. These people should have the opportunity to be heard. If you decide to gloss over or skip the rest of this chapter, no problem. It doesn't change the fact that Rick greatly helped more than 100 people. And it is certainly evidence that he can help you!

Hopefully, you will heed their words and get the help you need.

"Experiencing relief from pain is one of the greatest gifts a person can receive."

TESTIMONIALS *

NECK PAIN AND HEADACHES

"A peer introduced me to Rick. Before my appointment, I read his book on neck pain, to familiarize myself with his methods. When Rick assessed my shoulder and told me that my shoulder blades were too depressed, I was in total shock! My scapulae were not moving well, which caused my arm to literally move out of the socket and tear my cartilage. This was the first time anyone had ever assessed how my scapula moved in relation to my arm. This went against everything I had practiced/preached and focused on in my seven years of teaching Pilates! Shoulder blades down the back, long neck, but tons of shoulder pain with it!"
-Amazon Customer

"I read half the book and, even though Rick advises to read the whole thing before doing the exercises, well, I couldn't help myself ... I jumped right in. I did most of the exercises for the first time yesterday. Today I looked at a few of his online videos and did all of the exercises in the book. I can't believe how good my neck feels! It hasn't felt this loose and pain-free in many, many years ... as far back as I can remember, practically. The concept of my shoulders being responsible for neck pain simply never occurred to me and was never mentioned as a possibility when I tried to get help through chiropractors, massage therapists, ortho-bionomy practitioners, and acupuncturists. I really like the idea of helping myself, too.... Going to all these healthcare practitioners can get expensive and very frustrating when they don't "fix" you. I'm not a couch potato and I do stretching every day when I get up, but what with a couple of minor car accidents long ago and falling on our rocky terrain while hiking more than a few times, plus some bad posture habits, my whole body has gradually gotten so out of whack I didn't know where to start. Lately, I've been constantly gulping down ibuprofen due to almost constant headaches. My neck was at the very least chronically tense, but also usually quite stiff and sore. I'm looking forward to Rick's books that focus on hip problems and shoulder problems, because I need both of those, too! I've had an extremely painful shoulder for the past month or so due to too much time at the computer, I think. But the exercises in the neck pain book have helped this, as well. This book is extremely easy to read and understand. You're given a batch of exercises as well as helpful tips to follow during your daily routine. The videos Rick presents on his website are very clear and well executed." **-Amazon Customer**

"Perhaps the best part of buying this book was the fact that, when I emailed to ask the author about some exercises that I was having trouble completing, he responded right away!

*Any testimonial reference to a book is NOT referring to this book; rather, it is a reference to a previous book by Rick Olderman. However, this book presents the same exercises highlighted in the previous books.

Considering his very busy schedule, I was extremely grateful. We emailed back and forth, and he was amazingly kind to respond and recommend some additional therapies such as somatics, which is also on his website." **-Amazon Customer**

"I'm so impressed—this really works permanently! I was in a bad car accident that left me with a messed-up back and neck. After the accident, traditional doctors wanted to surgically put a metal rod in my back to straighten everything out; but I wanted to try a noninvasive path due to how active I am (I couldn't live with the restrictiveness of a rod). I went to a chiropractor for two years and then a physical therapist for two years trying to get rid of the pain. Over the years, I've been able to get my hips and ribs back into place, but I continued to have horrible neck pain and bad migraines. Nothing I was doing could get rid of terrible muscle spasms that would start in my shoulders and go all the way through the top of my head, which would then pull my neck vertebrae and my atlas out of place. I've had special work chairs ordered for my job, I've done dry needling, I've had massages, I've gotten my neck put into place 2–3 times a week, I've done neck strengthening exercises, I've had electricity therapy ... you name it, I've done it, but nothing worked to relieve pain for more than a couple of days. I'm very happy to say that this book has changed my life! I feel relief and I'm feeling well consistently! No more migraines, neck spasms, and countless doctor appointments. I was skeptical at first because the book reviews sounded too good to be true, but I'm here to say that everyone needs to give this a try—I've never felt so good since the car accident! Thank you, Rick Olderman, for this amazing resource." **-Amazon Customer**

"Between the book and the accompanying videos, this book is not only informative but goes into detail of what exercises should be done. I have had tight shoulder, neck, and head muscles along with nonstop headaches for the past three and a half years. I picked up this book recently after having it sit on a shelf way too long. I have spent a lot of money on copays and cash up front for drugs and medical procedures to rid me of my tight muscles and headaches. I think this book may actually work for me. I have been doing two of the exercises for almost a week now. I will slowly incorporate all of the exercises into my days and before or after I have gone for a run." **-Amazon Customer**

"I bought the knee and neck book because I have had chronic tension for many years. I like how the author treats the patient as

an intelligent being, and I appreciate that Olderman has the ability to put at times complex ideas in simple terms that anyone can understand. I used this book to understand what may be going on with my body and to be more informed when consulting a chiropractor or physical therapist rather than blindly following their recommendations."
-Amazon Customer

"In January of 2019, my primary care physician referred me to Rick's system. In two weeks, my neck issue was solved. Rick explained after my first diagnostic visit that my shoulder blades were stuck and that certain exercises would strengthen muscles so they would not 're-stick.' He also used pressure points and therapeutic massage to unstick the shoulders. I had so much hope that I actually did all the exercises Rick assigned and we proceeded to low back pain. With just a few more appointments and more work, the back pain was GONE. Then, we hit a wall. It concerned left foot pain that was so chronic and seemingly unsolvable that I never mentioned it to anyone. I just marched on slowly with a limp. Rick showed me that the arch in my left foot had completely fallen. In fact, the entire left side of my body was no longer weight-bearing. No wonder I have arthritis in my right knee. I got a picture of myself as an ostrich doing all the YARDWORK, the DOG WALKS, LAUNDRY, perched precariously on my right foot. So, Rick experimented over time with additions to my orthotics where the arch had fallen. He tried taping the right leg to take some stress off the right knee and added pads to the arch of the right orthotic, also. To encourage weight-bearing on the left side, I got a perfectly placed dose of cortisone in the arch of my left foot ... I stopped walking with a limp, so it was time to cast new orthotics with additional arch support on both sides, which Rick did. It worked! It's taken several months to develop strength in my left foot and leg but at last, it bears weight. My body is learning that it has a center of gravity and two sides with strength. At almost 73, I'm gardening again like a madwoman. I have an array of tools to use in the soil, and increased awareness of how to balance my body in motion. Thank you, Rick Olderman, and your system for the healing you bring so many people. Rick has published books addressing specific painful issues in different parts of the body called the *Fixing You* series. There is also a website: fixingyou.com. You'll want to view the videos the author provides to buyers of the book. It helps to see them done and have him explain them before you do them. You want to do them correctly so you won't hurt yourself and so you'll get all the benefits from them. He also shows modifications.

"The author does a good job of describing the anatomy of the shoulder and neck. He also explains why it's the shoulder causing your problems and not your neck. This is really the only book you need to get rid of that awful neck pain. Highly recommended." **-Susanna H**

"I've been diagnosed with a C3-C4 disk bulge and I'm suffering from neck and upper back pain and tension headaches for over six months. So far, I've been focusing on massages, neck traction, etc.; however, nothing helped me. Luckily, I found this book and realized that one of the root causes is a depressed shoulder caused by carrying a heavy backpack over one side and bad posture. After one week of exercise I already feel some improvements. Thank you, Rick, for this book and I hope to fix myself ASAP." **-Michael K**

"I like this book because it is short, has explanations that make sense, and gets you quickly to doing the exercises. I've gone for years with chronic migraines and have tried many different treatments, including medication, massage, acupuncture, and chiropractic. The only person to have explained that the muscles in my upper back were pulling on my neck was the chiropractor. When I read this book and saw that the physical therapist also talked a great deal about these particular muscles, I knew that I was finally on my way to neck pain relief. I didn't want to read a 300–400-page book on neck pain; I like this because it is concise, and the exercises can be done by anyone." **-Virginia**

"This book and the rest in the series are not only fantastic, but they come with a code to access videos which show the tests and the exercises. The visuals are great and are very helpful. I am a personal trainer with a passion to help others to age well and get rid of chronic pain and these books are great!" **-Shana L**

"At age 71, I had become resigned to a life with neck pain and headaches. I could not do normal chores like carrying groceries, vacuuming, laundry, or dog walks, without paying a huge price in pain. Deep tissue massages lasted a few days. Epsom salt baths and neck buddies heated in the microwave broke the worst bouts of pain. I pursued physical therapy for 14 years. Then, I got a referral to Rick's system. After a one-hour diagnosis, Rick Olderman pinpointed the issue: my shoulder blades were totally stuck. He gave me exercises to do for strengthening the muscles around the shoulder blades. Now, I can carry my groceries, vacuum, walk my dog, shovel snow, and sleep without neck pain. I'm going to have a whole new life of activity at 71. Wow!" **-Salle B**

"This book allows us 'real people' who don't have a medical degree to affect real change in our bodies. The author gives us information we can use and gives us the 'whys' behind it—but only if we want to know. I've already placed orders for the *Back Pain* book in this series—great gifts for friends and family." **-Virginia S**

"All of Rick Olderman's books are splendid. Aside from this one, I have one covering knees and hips and another for arms and shoulders. I find the exercises to be helpful."
-Amazon Customer

"This had information that I really needed when I hurt my neck. It agrees with other sources I have found." **-Amazon Customer**

"I had headaches for years and went to several doctors to try to solve the problem. I did lots of reading and research. After getting tired of having to rely on pills to take care of things, I went to a neurologist that suggested using the 'McKenzie' method (books available on Amazon). While I was looking at the McKenzie books, I also looked around for other books that might be highly rated and came across this one. Along with McKenzie, it pretty much did the trick! Now when I feel a headache coming on, I just get up from my chair in the office and do one of the stretches in this book, plus two from the McKenzie book. It almost always relieves the tension and my headache goes away, or at least doesn't progress to something that makes my work really difficult. On really rough days, I set my watch to beep every 30–45 minutes and do the stretches at those intervals. I hardly ever have to take any pills now. So, if you think you have headaches due to muscular tension, GET THIS BOOK. Seriously, it may solve your problem, and it costs way less than a doctor's visit!" **-Amazon Customer**

"The trick for us, I think, is to consciously keep in mind the couple of directions beneficial to us, all day long and every day, until they become natural." **-Kate**

"This book is wonderful! I have only recently started experiencing neck pain. Rick Olderman's insight into the possible association between shoulder posture and neck pain is amazing. Simple-to-understand, easy-to-do exercises to help alleviate neck pain. I would recommend it and am considering purchasing Olderman's book addressing elbow issues." **-Robin M**

"Thank you, Rick! It's a great book, and it gives you the facts in a straightforward manner, to figure out what is going on with your neck/shoulders. It gives just the right amount of medical background to answer the why and then great suggestions for answering the how! I have enjoyed the well-written steps to alleviate the pain, it has just enough graphics to help, and the videos online are the icing on the cake to make sure I can follow the exercises to the tee. The book was very well-written, to the point, and I found myself jumping in trying the exercises! I'm hooked and cannot wait to continue with the series." **-N Kazenske**

"Thank you so much! You're my hero. Your neck book has saved my life. I still haven't gotten to the exercises, but just correcting posture fixed 80% of my issues and has taken my headaches to almost none. I'm excited to work on the back next and then hip and knee (I was a childhood gymnast/ballerina)." **-Tina M**

"Before I launch into this review, I'd like to give some context to my comments, a frame for what follows about what I see as a remarkably helpful breakthrough approach to pain management and healing. As someone who has lived and worked in chronic pain (CP) since 1984 following a botched lumbar fusion (back) surgery, I think I've read more books and articles on the subject than I care to remember, many of them redundant, overly theoretical, or simply not helpful to me at all. So, I began this book with a jaded eye, a sort of 'show me something I don't know' mindset. But after reading and using two books in the *Fixing You* series by Rick Olderman, I felt compelled to spread the word so that more people might take advantage of this substantive yet practical handbook for dealing with specific pain areas. So here it goes: If you or someone you love is in CP (chronic pain), then you already know that long-term intractable pain—at any degree of intensity—is a totally different creature than episodic pain. In fact, in my own and many other CP sufferers' cases, what works well for most episodic pain simply does not work for long-term pain. In fact, what works with episodic pain (toothache, broken bone, etc.) when applied to chronic conditions often leads to a whole secondary set of problems. Narcotics are perhaps the best-known example of this compounding effect, for in chronic pain cases the dosage must be increased over time to provide the same relief. Then, unless guided by the holistic perspectives such as those of this book, so often CP (chronic pain) worsens and leads to depression, sleep disorders, anxiety, suicidal ideation and anger control difficulties, and more. It is a hell I would not wish on my worst enemy. For me, aside from the obvious benefit of exercises which work, the *Fixing You* series provides a way of thinking which can help the CP sufferer manage the pain and start on a healing process—all by a shift in how one experiences one's own body and movement. This is treated up front in the book(s) before even beginning the physical therapy aspect. The author makes it clear that each person is responsible for their own healing, that how they visualize themselves and how they think about their pain has a direct impact on how well the physical therapy exercises do their healing work.

"For me the takeaways of the book are as follows:

1. You own your own healing process, self-awareness may be difficult when racked with pain, but it will be the key to fixing yourself.
2. Focus on your whole person and not the pain site itself (again, not an easy task).
3. When it comes to healing the body, function trumps structure, meaning that a structural defect on your MRI need not be a final verdict. Rick Olderman's solutions lie in teaching the body more ergonomically correct postures and movement, optimizing the body's innate ability to heal itself.

"Another valuable bonus of the *Fixing You* book series is that you can access videos online via a password-access website provided when you purchase the book. The style of writing is personable and clear, void of preaching or philosophical verbiage which can often muddle rather than clarify. With these books a CP sufferer has a better understanding of what they must think—as well as do—to truly fix themselves. Even if your pain is not in the neck or back, this is a must-read for all with chronic pain. Perhaps the biggest problem I have with this book is that Rick is not down the street so I can visit him when I need to! I give this book five stars!" **-Dana L**

"For the past fifteen years and increasingly, I suffered what I thought were high blood pressure–related headaches. It finally occurred to me that my headaches were possibly related to a 35-year-old rugby injury, a separated clavicle. I found Rick's book and within days was headache- and neck pain–free. I had a slight relapse having slackened the exercise regimen but will not make that mistake again. My shoulder has more flexibility now and feels stronger. I've been doing yoga assiduously for twenty years, but those postures did not address the problem of my lowered shoulder blade; Rick's exercises do. Whether Rick's program works for your shoulder/neck/headache problem(s), I do not know, but the book is inexpensive, and the program is not too physically demanding. It may be worthwhile to give it a try. I am now without what had been near-chronic pain, for which I am most grateful." **-Amazon Customer**

"I have been having severe headaches and neck pain. This book has given me many tips and exercises to use. They have been very helpful so far." **-T Morris**

"This book has great information and is very easy to understand! The videos are great, and the exercises are unique! Rick has tons of knowledge! He really likes to help people and he does! I'm feeling much better already! Don't sleep on your tummy! Great advice! I highly recommend this book to everyone who wants to live pain-free!" **-Alejo M**

"I cannot recommend this book enough! If you suffer with a stiff neck, headaches, or shoulder pain, then get yourself this book. Following a 4-year ankle injury, meaning I spent most of my time looking down to watch for uneven ground, I started looking for a way to help with my constant neck and shoulder pain, as I was concerned with all the painkillers necessary to function. I always read the reviews of self-help books, as there are quite a lot of poorly informed guides and was a bit dubious about the fact that there were no UK reviews for this product. The reviews from Amazon.com were gushing and as it is quite reasonably priced, I thought I'd risk it. THANK GOODNESS I DID!

"The advice in it is great: technical without being too scientific, plus easy to follow. Honestly, within 2 days of doing the exercises I could feel my whole neck and shoulder loosening up. The anatomical information at the beginning of the book gave me a clear image in my mind of what part of my body I should be focused on during each exercise. There is even a link to videos of Rick showing you each exercise to help you to really make sure you're on the right track. It's a very comprehensive book.

"The retraining of my muscles did cause some soreness at first, but I would encourage you to persevere through this as two weeks after doing the program each evening, I only need to adjust my posture and stretch my scapula a little when I feel the old pain creep in during the day and it's gone! Give this book a go and you won't be disappointed."
-Amazon Customer

"Rick's system was fantastic! From my first visit to graduating, they were extremely attentive, insightful, and patient. I would highly recommend the book and will be back for any future injuries. My doctor recommended surgery, but through physical therapy, I was back to myself within six weeks. Amazing!"
-Eden E

"I love this book. It is short, easy to read, and has immediately useful suggestions on how to deal with headaches and neck pain. I am a physical therapist and a Pilates Instructor who is always looking for ways to help my clients. This book is a gem. I have found it to be a useful tool in helping people understand concepts I studied while getting my master's.... You do not have to have an anatomy or biomechanical background to understand Rick's book. He makes understanding human movement fun and gives people the gift of comprehending how movement works. I recommend this and all the *Fixing You* series to those in pain and those who want to understand more about the human body and how it moves." **-M Martin**

"I am so grateful for this book and for Rick. My head pain has improved so much!" **-K King**

"The first time I did the exercises which were simple and easy to do, I went to bed pain-free, amazing. I'm not very good at sticking to an exercise routine but when you see such good results it keeps you going. The video clips on the website show you exactly how to do them properly. He gives you a lot of tips and advice in the book which really makes you think about the way you move, the position you sleep in, your posture when driving. Things that I had never thought about. I would highly recommend this book." **-Geraldine**

"I came across this book by accident whilst searching for something else and after reading other reviews thought I'd give it a go. I've never written a product review before, but this is the most useful book I've ever bought! I've had severe neck pain and headaches for over 20 years, been through all the usual treatments—physio, chiropractor, osteopath, etc., plus various medications—and nothing has worked. As I read through the early chapters learning more about how the neck and shoulders work and feeling where various muscles were, I could already feel a difference in how my neck felt, how changing my posture released some of the pressure on my neck. When sitting down to read the book I had the usual pounding headache that starts after a few hours at work, but an hour after finishing the early chapters the pain was easing—without the aid of painkillers!! I've made huge efforts to follow the first couple of exercises in the book and change my usual posture and have now gone a week without a headache and with minimal discomfort in my neck—I am completely sold on the book and will now be working towards some of the other exercises in the hope that eventually I will cure my neck pain."
-Amazon Customer

FOOT AND ANKLE

"I started out with this book and loved it so much I had to get all the *Fixing You* books. I love how it explains everything so that it is easy to understand plus the exercises to fix the issue are a bonus. My right shoulder bothers me on and off but since I read and followed the instructions in the book it has not given me any issues. As a massage therapist, these books have been beyond helpful to me in the anatomy areas." **-J Mulcahy**

"My therapist is terrific, but my pain persisted after the acute injuries were 'solved.' I was afraid this pain was a lifelong sentence. I followed Rick's instructions about analyzing one's gait. I then walked down the hall at home pain-free albeit taking small steps as advised. I'm back to a full shift in the Emergency Dept. My husband will help me test my femur alignment today. I hope to be back hiking very soon!" **-Kathleen S**

"I've had problems with pronation in my right foot for years and this book is finally helping me figure out how to take care of it. The author talks about all kinds of foot issues: possible causes, the relationship of the foot to the calf, knee, and hip, how to 'walk better,' how to tape your foot or ankle (amazing for pain relief), how to loosen up your feet, pronation, supination, bunions, hammer toes, and so on. Over the years, I've been to several physical therapists and podiatrists. I've tried custom and customized orthotics that, at best, kept the foot from getting worse, but never improved my foot to be comfortable enough to walk barefoot. In other words, the foot never changed. This book will show you how to change things in your feet so they will function normally again. Another great big thanks to the author! (I also have the hip book which helped me get rid of a very stubborn and annoying problem with my SI joint.)"
-Amazon Customer

"I rolled my ankle back in March of 2018 and noticed pain in my knee about 7–8 months later as I slowly got back into hiking shape. Going downhill was becoming an issue and I also started noticing soreness while at rest. I moved to Colorado to hike so I was worried that my injury was going to prevent me from hiking and/or get worse over time. Physical therapy not only got rid of both the soreness and ankle pain but also has generally helped my hiking—doing more miles now than I was before my initial injury and with no pain!"**-Brennan G**

"I ordered this book out of curiosity, but also because I, myself, have ankle pain. I already had the book about back pain from Olderman, but since I liked it and thought that book was very informative, I decided to order this book too. I have started reading the *Foot & Ankle Pain* book and have started with some exercises. The pain in my ankle does not fully cease, but the exercises make it feel better."
-Amazon Customer

"This is a really great book with practical self-help advice to resolve chronic conditions. This book has helped me to look at my foot and ankle issues from a different perspective and the advice in the books is worth the cover price alone. You also get bonus access to video tutorials on his website. This brings the information to life. It really feels like Rick is sharing his valuable knowledge." **-Jack R**

"I have employed the exercises in a couple of Rick Olderman's books—he does an excellent job of providing the right level of detail to enable me to successfully do the exercises myself. I highly recommend these books." **-Jon F**

"This book has lots of information. I never taped my feet, but this book convinced me to. It shows you how. It worked well for me. You cannot do this if you are diabetic so talk to your doctor first. The author also recommends taking smaller steps and explains why in detail. This helped also." **-Amazon Customer**

"I came for therapy very sore on 7-15-19. I completed therapy on 8-12-19. Therapy took the pain away and I can now do daily walks and am also back to playing golf." **-Ed W**

"Rick's system did a great job helping me recover from foot surgery. He understood my goals were not just to heal but to get back to doing the things I enjoy. In just three months, I went from pain, discomfort, and swelling to an almost full recovery and level of activity. He taught me lots of helpful exercises and stretches which I will continue to use." **-Melinda P**

"It was very well-written and easy to understand. I am flat-footed and I have trouble with my ankle. Now that I understand the mechanics of the foot and ankle, I know what to do and not to do. I have bought other books from this series and have never been disappointed." **-Amazon Customer**

"This is a great book for anyone who still has some pain after they have read the author's hip/knee pain book. You do need someone else to help you with some of the exercises as the author states, so this book was not as beneficial for me as the hip/knee book, but this is still a great book!" **-J Bell**

"When I started working with Rick's system, I was just starting to awkwardly walk again, with pain in several spots, and couldn't do much else. Over the course of a few months, I was able to eliminate those pain points, slowly start hiking again, get back into the gym, and finally start climbing 13ers and 14ers again and get back to my usual active lifestyle. Looking forward to skiing again this winter with my new titanium tibia." **-Mike V**

HIP AND KNEE

"I've been suffering from progressively worsening hip pain for a couple of years now, which I've been pretty sure is due to a muscular imbalance— 'gluteal amnesia'—caused by sitting too much. There's lots of advice out there on YouTube and in books that claim to tell you what's wrong and how to fix it, but none of them even came close to helping me or allowing me to definitively figure out the exact nature of the malfunction. So, I was pretty skeptical (but desperate) when I purchased this *Fixing You* book on relieving hip and knee pain, but I am so glad I took a chance on another PT who claimed to be able to help."
-Amazon Customer

"I read the book and took it to heart. Very helpful for recovery from hip replacement and tendonitis caused by PT aggravating a prior glute injury! It's very helpful to have the online video component as I am very visual. It's definitely a great program."
-Amazon Customer

"Yes, it will take some work and effort on your part to achieve relief, but these are things you certainly can do, without an unreasonable expenditure of time and effort. I've only been doing the exercises for a few days and can already feel a difference. Best of all, now that I know exactly what's going on with the muscles involved, I feel very motivated and confident that I'll be able to work through the problem on my own.

"I still think this book is great—it made me aware of how muscle imbalances can really mess with your joints but do yourself a favor and seek a professional diagnosis sooner than later ... So don't be stubborn and think you can fix things all by yourself, especially if you are older—seek hands-on help and a firm diagnosis sooner than later." **-Amazon Customer**

"I tore my lateral meniscus over Christmas break. I could barely walk. I saw an orthopedic surgeon and he suggested I see a PT instead of surgery. I saw Rick and after the first appointment I felt so much better. I slowly recovered, doing the exercises Rick gave me. He not only helped me heal from my injury but addressed old patterns in my posture and walking that caused the injury. I feel great and would recommend Rick's system wholeheartedly." **-Holly H**

"When I came to Rick Olderman, I had been suffering with elbow pain for about 8 or 9 months. I thought I would get better through rest. My progress was very slow. Rick gave me stretching and exercise routines that gave me dramatic improvement in the reduction of my elbow pain. During my elbow recovery, I injured my hip. He incorporated the routines to help my hip recover in just a few weeks. I feel extremely thankful for his therapy and genuine concern for my well-being. I know if I had not come to see him, I would still be dealing with significant pain." **-David M**

"In a word, this book is fantastic! Rick Olderman not only enabled me to match my pain with a diagnosis (anterior pelvic tilt on the right side) but also goes into detail about how to fix it and how to correct bad habits that caused the muscular imbalance in the first place. The book taught me about the anatomy relevant to hip and knee problems yet was easy to understand." **-Amazon Customer**

"I had both of my knees replaced this year, the left in April and the right in September. I had quite a bit of pain with my first knee replacement, but Rick's system really helped me through it. A past chiropractor had diagnosed me with a shortened right leg. But when we did measurements, it was that my pelvis was out of whack and got me totally aligned! When I had my right knee done in September, it was so easy. I was up without any cane or anything, two weeks postop!" **-Karen B**

"When I first came to see Rick, I had a sharp pain in my right knee when I climbed the stairs. Rick diagnosed my problem as weak glutes, a tracking problem in my right leg, and a gait in which I locked my leg with every step. Rick had me do several exercises which strengthened my glutes and my legs and improved my balance. My knee pain disappeared within a week or two and I am completely without pain now. I also feel stronger and more balanced. I continue to do the exercises Rick recommended and I continue to improve. Thanks, Rick!" **-James W**

"I had a remote left knee injury and had been struggling with chronic pain due to patellofemoral syndrome, worsening once the birth of my children. Physical therapy identified some easy changes that I could integrate into my everyday life, without having to spend lots of time on a cumbersome daily routine. I am now able to sit in a movie theater and take flights without days of left knee pain following." **-Kara A**

"I originally came to Rick's system after straining my MCL in a ski accident. Rick and Tayler were awesome in helping me with understanding the entire picture of what was happening. Through the process, they identified issues with my ankle as well. It has been a huge gift to learn more about my body and to be self-aware. I'm grateful for your work and desire to help! Thanks!" **-Jeff T**

"I found some exercises in this book that made my hip feel good immediately, after four years of PT, massage, negative MRIs, and X-rays. The exercises section with photos is easy to understand." **-Amazon Customer**

"Years of excruciating lower back pain from all types of physical activity eventually led to a severe lower back strain. The next year of self-treatment had little effect so eventually I came to Body in Balance Physical Therapy for professional help. Within a single treatment,

I was shown that I had been hyperextending my knees while walking/standing my entire life. Through the exercises and postural changes, I not only recovered from my strain but made vast improvements in my overall back/leg strength and pain." **-Nevell G**

"This book was extraordinarily helpful. Olderman lays out the anatomy involved in a thorough but simple way so that I could visualize what needed to be strengthened, what needed to be stretched, and why. He then talks about normal movement patterns—walking, sitting, etc.—and how you're going to shift these as you retrain your muscles. This is such an important part, because, of course, walking happens several thousand times in a day, and if you shift that, it has even more effect than the exercises that you'll do maybe once per day. The exercises are not numerous which is cool because too many exercises make things too tedious.

"I had labral tears in my hip about eight years ago, with two arthroscopic surgeries on the same hip. I've been trying rehab ever since, with the help of several highly qualified physical therapists. I wish I'd been given this book at the beginning of that process because it really clarifies the problems and the goals nicely. This book is an easy read; I think I read it in two or three sittings. The book gives you access to video tapes of each of the exercises plus a few other useful tips. Highly recommended for hip problems. Olderman's explanation of how the entire leg functions and how its joints interact in walking is more graspable than anything else I've read on this topic. And I've read quite a bit, believe me (Oh, pain is such a motivator...)." **-Amazon Customer**

"I am a distance runner who has been battling injuries since 2010. I practically gave up on running when my friend introduced me to this book. I hate reading but I was desperate, and this book wasn't a thick textbook, so I decided to give it a try. This book is very easy to read, and yes, he does use a lot of terminology but there's no escaping that if you want to sound professional! I never knew how important strong glutes can be for preventing knee pain and ever since reading this book, my life has changed. At the same time, I'm also seeing a physical therapist to help enforce some of the things I've learned in this book (I had him show me a bunch of other glute strengthening exercises) and after two weeks of absolutely no running, followed by some strength training and PT visits, I'm now back up to five miles of pain-free running. I hope to be back to half marathon distances by the end of summer and maybe marathon distances in 2014. Wish me luck..." **-Amazon Customer**

"Have you gone to the doctor and were told that one leg is shorter than the other? And you thought, 'how in the world did my leg shrink?' Most likely your hip is out of alignment and the whole problem is muscular. You may be prescribed a heel lift that supposedly fixes everything, but it may make things worse, because now you're adding another issue for your body to deal with, and it may even pull out your hip even more (like in my case).

"This book explains what's happening with your hips, has some good drawings to explain the issue and some simple exercises. I've had this hip issue (and knee problems) for years and I tried all kinds of stuff, including physical therapy, yoga, Pilates, etc. This book is what finally took me from frustration to healing. Make no mistake, your hip may be out because of bad habits or from an injury, and the longer you've lived with your problem, the longer it will take to get better. But don't give up! It's so worth it! Besides, what's the alternative...

"The hardest thing about the healing process is to get rid of bad habits like crossing your legs or standing on one leg, slouching in the chair, sitting uneven, etc. But this book will help you identify those and give you positive reinforcement that you can actually fix yourself. A big thank you to the author!" **-Mary**

"I found this book very useful. I had numerous knee issues and most of the physical therapists couldn't pinpoint the reason. I finally found some therapists and a chiropractor that were able to diagnose and help me, but this book was very helpful because I could understand what they were talking about and because I could ask them the right questions.

"The genius of this book lies in its simplicity, and I think the author has done a great job presenting complex ideas in layman's terms. I realized I had a rotated hip, which I am able to fix, but my knee pain has persisted. Using this book, I realized that I also have femoral retroversion. No physical therapist told me this or paid attention to it, but now I feel like I can talk to them, tell them I have this, and ask for treatment for that. I have now ordered the neck and shoulder book and hope to resolve those issues as well with the help of the exercises and explanations in that book."

-Amazon Customer

"I like to consider myself a long-distance runner; however, I've noticed that I couldn't get any relief in my knee when running. I started physical therapy again as I felt that I knew it could help me. During physical therapy, I learned many exercises to help stretch my muscles, as my body gained strength. Now I am given the tools to stretch my muscles and also conversation of nutrition and how that is very important." **-Melanie A**

"All of the *Fixing You* books are excellent. I have three and am constantly looking at one or another, depending on what ailment I have at any given time. He has excellent expertise in these body parts and what makes them tick. Boy, do I wish I could sit in a room with him and go over all this with him!!! He's my one and only go-to for these issues that keep popping up now that I am older. Don't know what I would do without his excellent books!"

-Amazon Customer

"This book really helped me reduce my knee and hip pain. I was just hitting dead ends when it came to regular doctors. I figured it must be a muscular problem rather than a bone problem and this book confirmed that it was indeed muscular. I did have MRIs to rule out structural/joint/bone dysfunctions though. The book is easy to read, especially if you're not familiar with anatomy terms. The author explains concepts in an easy-to-understand manner. I did need further assistance from a physical therapist who specializes in sports injuries due to other issues, but this book got me on the path and helped decrease my pain considerably. I would suggest it to anyone who has knee/hip issues, especially if nothing else seems to be working in your favor. Definitely a great help and for a lot less than a copay or doctor's visit!" **-Amazon Customer**

"Although many of the reviews do state that it may be somewhat simplistic, I do not disagree with them. It can be, but still quite informative. Also, without reiterating most of what he explains, would cut down on the size of it as well. I have been suffering from nagging back issues for some time and since I have been running, I have had hip and knee issues. This helped me locate my issue and present it in an easy-to-understand format. It has only been a week since I have gotten and read the book, so it is too soon to tell how effective it is for me personally, but I do highly recommend this to anyone if they do suffer from any level of pain and want to be able to have self-empowerment. Doctors can use so much jargon and still not help you understand what is wrong and if you will improve. That is where Rick Olderman and this book steps in."

-Amazon Customer

"Out of the four or five hip and knee pain treatment books that I've ordered from Amazon, this one is by far the best. The author spends a good deal of time explaining the causes of hip and knee pain, so that when you undertake the exercises he suggests, you do so with some understanding of what you are doing and why. He clearly places the burden of 'fixing yourself' on the patient, making it clear that not only must he do the exercises suggested, but that he must do them CORRECTLY and with awareness. And they work! After a couple of weeks, my hip pain has markedly decreased ... and I can now go to bed without three ice bags and a Vicodin to get me through the night!"

-Amazon Customer

"My nine-year-old daughter sustained a left knee bone bruise following a fall in gym class at school. This injury also caused her muscles to tighten up around her left knee. Tori was scared and frustrated, unable to participate in her active lifestyle full of bike riding, walking, hiking, skiing, horseback riding, and gymnastics. Tori began physical therapy with Rick in March with high hopes of healing. She and Rick worked very hard together. He guided Tori in a calm and confident manner. Tori learned that she was going to heal fully if she continued to put forth great effort at home with the exercises Rick assigned. She did! Tori is so proud of herself. I (her mother) am so proud of her and so happy with the guidance Rick gave her to get to this point. Tori is back at all her typical activities, all thanks to Rick's hard work and Tori's determination. Thank you." **-Michelle R**

"Love this book. It's easy to understand and the exercises are easy to follow. Viewing the videos makes you realize how long you have been mistreating your body. Believe it or not but I experienced some relief after doing just one set of each exercise. I was told one leg was shorter than the other and thanks to Rick I found out that was not the case. No surgery for me. GET THE BOOK if you are in pain." **-Maureen T**

"From this book I learned how certain standing, sitting, and walking habits can grind away cartilage and weaken muscles and joints. By using the movement guidelines presented in this book, my joints feel better and the muscles around the hip and knee joints feel stronger, taking some stress away from the bones." **-M Benson**

"I purchased this book several months ago because of episodic bouts of hip pain. I found the book to be very thorough in content of hip and knee problems and exercises to improve the condition. It was not until recently that I began doing the exercises regularly. The exercises are very helpful, and my hip pain has diminished considerably. I can walk without limping. The book is written with such clarity and accompanying visuals are very helpful." **-Dr. Florence Ouzts**

"I first came to Rick's system in January 2019 in so much pain I was seriously contemplating quitting my yoga teaching job. Since February 2018 I had been going to doctors and physical therapists trying to get a proper diagnosis. Finally, my primary care doctor referred me to Rick and his team. Over the next six months working with Rick, we figured it out, the injury and treatment plan. Every session seemed to bring us more clarity. Rick was as dedicated (if not more!) as me to get this puzzle solved. Using a combination of exercise, taping, dry needling, and a splint we got there! By June I was back to walking, jogging, cycling, and my full schedule of yoga. And the best part was going from constant pain to a pain level of zero. I can't thank Rick enough!" **-Deborah B**

"For the past couple of decades, my life has been increasing pain and limping. I have had two surgeries on my knee including replacement. I have also had six-plus years of postural corrective therapy. I have improved but still not a normal functional gait. Since I was still looking for answers, I came across this book. It described the problems I have had and the muscle weakness that was the cause. It is unbelievable to me that this was missed by so many health professionals. I have purchased three of Rick's books and have found helpful suggestions in each of them. I highly recommend this book and the videos are very helpful. My life has turned around in a very hopeful direction." **-Thomas C**

"This book is well-written and to the point. What he says makes complete sense (coming from a veteran critical care RN). I am very thankful for this information and grateful to the writer. I was able to determine the cause of my knee pain and have already seen improvement from the one exercise that I have incorporated into my daily life: 'walk the walk.' Also, I have learned that my body mechanics were way off. Do not have any invasive procedures without doing all that you can first. Draining fluid from your knees is a lifelong procedure. It always fills right back up unless you get to the root of the problem." **-Amazon Customer**

"I was introduced to Rick Olderman's *Fixing You* books via an Amazon recommendation. After reading a few paragraphs using the 'Look Inside' feature, I decided to give the book a try. I'm hoping to improve some symptoms from standing on one leg over time. A few things I'd like to share about the book:

1. The book is based on current medical research. It is very easy to read. The concepts make a lot of common sense.
2. The anatomy introduced in the book is very informative and not too hard to understand. I felt I got enough information to get on the right track of self-help.
3. Rick pointed out some very common problems people have with a couple simple case studies. I once considered the issues unique to me. Now I realize that my case is typical among people of many different trades. And my issues have been corrected successfully.
4. Rick included some simple and effective exercises that really work. Besides verbal explanation and illustrations, he also loaded some online videos for people who purchased the book. This eliminated lots of guesswork and errors when doing the exercises.

"I highly recommend Rick's book. If you're reading this review, you owe it to yourself to get the book." **-Amazon Customer**

"There are very clear explanations of hip mechanics. There are simple exercises which are very well explained. After two years with pain and trying everything, and it is after following the recommended exercises that I have started to get better." **-Esperanza C**

"I have a pelvis inclined on the left and rotating backward. I have a sole in my left shoe, had sessions with a physiotherapist and my unbalance was still increasing. Surprisingly, the book was hard to find on Amazon.fr despite the fact it's the only one I know for the moment to treat that specific hip imbalance. It filled my lack of knowledge on basic anatomy and biomechanics with multiple and simple visuals. It provided corrective exercises. After a few weeks, I can already see improvements, but I have no illusion, it's long-term rehab after years of bad patterns." **-Amazon Customer**

"I did a lot of searching on the internet to understand the physical makeup of the hips to try and understand why my hips hurt all the time and it was frustrating and not really very informative. Then I found this book, and it all made sense. It's well illustrated, uses simple non-technical terms, and includes exercises that make sense. I've been recommending it to all my friends that have the same issues." **-J Ellis**

"What a wonderful book! The exercises are simple and easily done daily, and the relief from hip pain that I felt was almost immediate. Walking in the woods with my dogs has become a pleasure, rather than an activity undertaken with trepidation (I have to go regardless, my dogs wouldn't hear of anything else). If your hips or knees hurt, get this book!"
-Amazon Customer

"This series of books is excellent, there is a self-diagnostic scheme which enables you to find out where the trouble comes from, and there are simple exercises to correct your problems. On his site there are free-access videos (the access code is in the book), and you can also download them for a modest sum. I emailed the author, and he answered the same day. What more can you want?" **-Amazon Customer**

Excellent book! I finally understood the underlying cause of my hip and knee pain. Clear explanation and illustration of muscle and bone movements involving the hip and knee. The suggestions for change of habits really worked for me and so did the exercises." **-Ella F**

"All of Rick Olderman's books are practical and accessible for the layperson and for the professional. As a massage therapist, I must keep my practice 'within the scope' of massage therapy. However, what Rick communicates in these volumes is something I can suggest my clients investigate. The online videos are excellent, too." **-Amazon Customer**

"The exercises in this book worked a miracle for my knee. Within a couple of weeks, I am almost completely pain-free. I highly recommend this book." **-Amazon Customer**

"Having been diagnosed with the necessity of two replacement knees and hips, due to osteoporosis and arthritis joints, I decided to investigate alternatives, and I have learned much from investigation and reading books like this. No operations to date and none planned. I think I have been listed as 'NC,' non-compliant, but if I can strengthen the muscles, tendons, and ligaments which are part responsible for the movement at these joints, that is what I intend to do. I have found this and other books so helpful, far different from the consultant who just said, 'four operations, you will be out of action for two years,' I have supplemented these books with physiotherapy and osteopathy privately because I have not had surgery. I am not eligible under the NHS for this funding, although I have paid into the system for many years! Buy this book and others, read and use the information, the only Magic Wand is Yourself!" **-Amazon Customer**

"The exercises in this book are clear, easy to follow, and effective if practiced daily. From a code in the back of the book one can access online videos of the exercises that are helpful for people who may not be used to following this kind of instruction. I highly recommend this for people with bad knees."
-Amazon Customer

"Excellent book. This was an Amazon suggestion that came when I was trying to find appropriate exercises to help ease severe hip and knee pain. Rick Olderman explained the mechanics of the problem and his exercises have enabled me to regain lost muscle and realign a rotated and tilted pelvis. It is important to be committed to the regular daily exercises both physically and mentally."
-Amazon Customer

"Olderman has done it again. This is the third book in his series that I have read. I used his neck book and by correcting my posture I got rid of 80% of my chronic neck pain from the last 26 years. I have already started changing the way I walk and stand, focusing on my glutes and hips. I am confident that the knee pain that I've had from childhood gymnastics will soon disappear. Thanks, Rick, for pain-free living—at last!" **-Amazon Customer**

"Rick Olderman has great insight as to how our bodies work and should not work in the third book of his *Fixing You* series. By following his simple explanations on why we have pain in our hips and knees, you will completely heal yourself. I have passed on Rick's advice to many of my students who have had back, neck, hip, or knee problems, knowing I am giving advice that will ultimately improve their golfing experience. Keep them coming, Rick!"
-Mel S

"This book has excellent advice on improving how you handle your walking, so you injure your hip less." **-Aisjah H**

LOWER BACK

"I had two issues going on at the same time: a bulging disc at L4 and L5 and a narrowing artery in my left leg, which stopped me from walking more than a few hundred feet. I had an angioplasty which opened the artery and now I could address the back pain. The exercises in this book are doing what an orthopedic surgeon, neurosurgeon, and cortisone shots could not do, and that is to relieve my back pain. I have been doing the exercises recommended every morning for the past four days and I could not believe these simple exercises (Trapezius Release, Back Arch series, Tummy Arching) could relieve the back pain from a bulging disc, but they did. I have been using my cell phone to watch the videos on his website while I am on the floor (cushioned pad) learning the exercises. It has really helped in learning how to position your body so that you feel the muscle contractions Rick is instructing you to feel. I will be adding additional exercises as I master the technique for each one. Thank you, Rick Olderman, for your ability to transfer your knowledge to others. I am so grateful." **-Barbara G**

"I've always been a physical person. I created and tended 9 flower beds by the time I was nine years old. On the tennis team in high school, I wore out a pair of Converse tennis shoes every two weeks. I had scoliosis in my spine and was always a bit stiff. Low back pain was always tough for me, so on my 40th birthday, I could hardly get out of bed. Then I got older and a tennis injury from high school was turning walks into nightmares. Every step hurt. Back pain persisted but wasn't as bad as the left foot pain. The right knee was taking all the weight that the left foot couldn't handle, and it started hurting a lot! There was a huge stop sign across most of the things I loved to do—at only age 72. Then my doctor referred me to Rick Olderman Physical Therapy. For the first time, I was honest about how many body parts HURT! Rick solved my neck pain so quickly that we got a referral for the other three problems. He kept experimenting with additions to my orthotics for several weeks till we had it right. Then he cast entirely new orthotics. My feet love the new support and the balance the orthotics provide. Back pain is gone. The right knee is fifty percent better since it no longer must do all the work. Thank you, Rick, for getting me back in balance.... The stop sign has been removed. I now get to do all the favorite things I want to do with my 72-year-old body." **-Sallie B**

"I had awful back pain. Rick spoke with confidence, knowledge, and encouragement. I followed his guidelines and now know how to keep healthy, long-term. Thanks for all your help. We are lucky you have such a passion." **-Margaret P**

"I always wondered why when I walked, I drifted to the left. I found out that is because my femur bone turned outward from flaying my legs outward when sitting as a kid. I have a difficult time sitting cross-legged. He

suggested turning the right foot out helped so much. I have had far less problems with my back bothering me. I cannot believe one simple adjustment made such a difference."
-Amazon Customer

"I came for PT with back pain, leg weakness, and balance problems. After working with Rick, my back pain has resolved and I'm gaining strength in my legs. Rick has given me many tools to continue in my progress. I'm very happy with the results. Thank you so much, Rick." **-Rebecca F**

"I have the first edition too. Rick has added more exercise illustrations and links to helpful videos in this new edition. If you want the WHY your back hurts, this is the only book that will tell you not only how to fix the pain, but why it hurts. Doesn't matter if it's an old injury, or you've already had back surgery, or some other excuse, Rick will help you to feel better. He saved me from being an invalid because of pain when physiatrists, physical therapists, and doctors could not help at all. (I did not want surgery because if you do the research, you will find it doesn't always help the pain, doesn't deal with the causes of the pain, and sometimes makes the pain worse).

"Rick and his book have been outstanding in helping me with back issues. Most of all I appreciate what a great medical and patient advocate he is. I highly recommend the book."
-JC

"Great illustrations, easy-to-understand instructions. My best back pain book."
-Amazon Customer

"I would highly recommend this book. My son bought me the hip and knee book for my birthday, I have since ordered all of Mr. Olderman's books. In fact, my husband and I went to see him just this week, and he is very intelligent and kind. He has given us exercises to do and helped us out by diagnosing what we specifically need to work on. You won't regret buying this book and trying it out."
-Amazon Customer

"I had crippling sciatica from a desk job, commute, and decades of competitive volleyball. I was scheduled for a hip replacement (two years ago now). First, Rick was the first to troubleshoot this as a hip problem (which led to back issues). Obviously, my arthritic hip is still a problem, but it is minor and solved with Aleve. The book gave me great visuals, demystified some of the body parts and how they work together, and gave me some very simple but effective stretches and tips to put off my surgery while living a pain-free life. My hip is damaged, and will fix eventually, but all the negative impact surrounding my back is solved with some easy routine stretches." **-Carrie E**

"This book is truly amazing because of the simplicity with which it explains the various musculoskeletal behaviors. Rick has nailed down the balance of being technical and yet explaining things in an easy way. The accompanying videos (links to his website) are very clear and help in carrying out the tests and exercises in a proper way. I chanced upon this after more than 6 months of living with the sciatic pain resulting from bulged discs in the lower back. The physiotherapy has helped me make remarkable progress in the past 6 weeks. I was drawn to this book as I still had some unanswered questions. I struggled to understand why my gluteal sciatic pain would still persist despite some very good physiotherapy. Rick provides such a lucid explanation of things with easy-to-follow tests. It made me realize certain seemingly minor corrections that I needed to make in my standing, sitting, and walking posture could have such a profound impact on my situation. Using these tests, I was also able to acutely reduce the problems that I had been having. I have started following the remedial exercises. It's still early days, but it does look like it has answered some of the persistent problems. Even if the book is not able to help me get over my problem completely, it's worth a read to understand what harm I had been causing to the body through seemingly negligible postural habits." **-K Sehmi**

"I was a little skeptical at first, but after reading the first few chapters of the book, it gives you the science behind why you are having pain in your back. Then I tried the stretches and exercises and after a week or so I started to feel the difference. Slowly the pain started to dissipate, and now I am pain-free. If you are on the fence about buying this book, I am here to tell you that you will not regret it. Believe me when I tell you that I was just as undecided as you are, but I finally said: nothing ventured, nothing gained. What are you waiting for, order the book." **-Judith P**

"I can recommend this book to those who want to understand how their body works and develop an awareness of the movements that give rise to pain, without resorting to painkillers or surgery. Armed with the information in the book and the free videos, you are able to adapt your movements to alleviate pain. I suffered from severe sciatica, but by understanding the movements that had been causing the pain and using the simple tips and exercises, the condition improved so much that it's given me the confidence to know that I can now deal with the problem myself should it recur." **-Pauline W**

"'The Sherlock Holmes of solving body pain puzzles,' Dr. Rick Olderman, shares the frustrations, failures, and triumphs of his journey to discover why we have pain. I have always said that this man is a genius. Now I see that his ability to help others fix their pain is 99% perseverance! What a heart to help others. Having purchased a dozen of his books for myself and others over the last 15 or so years, I can testify that everything he says is accurate. He has answered my questions via email, sometimes almost immediately! I am 75 years old and know how to walk, sit, stand, move my neck, shoulders, hips, etc. without pain. Thanks, Dr. Rick! You've hit this one out of the ballpark!" **-Amazon Customer**

"Rick has been the most significant provider in a long journey toward healing my physical ailments. He was able to help me after multiple other providers were not. I felt like giving up, but luckily didn't and reached out to the right person, Rick, who has been my champion, tirelessly supporting with positivity and encouragement, while challenging me to overcome negative habits of using/misusing my body and pushing me when it was needed to be consistent with my strength training. What also made a difference is that Rick has an extremely impressive knowledge and the most up-to-date understanding of the body. His techniques are vast and highly progressive. In fact, his vast repertoire, keen observational ability, and invaluable insights are what made him stand out among other providers where they all were eventually stymied. He took my puzzling condition as an exciting challenge to figure out. He was targeted and quick in his assessments, and in a fairly short period of time, he was able to identify and effectively treat what had been a previously mysterious condition. He is always present, prompt, and thoughtful—a fantastic communicator and listener, working collaboratively while inspiring/motivating with endless positivity. My treatment experience has been amazing in every way, and I am pain-free, stronger, and feeling better than I thought was possible. I can now enjoy activities that I haven't been able to in years and never feel weighed down by physical issues. I am eternally grateful to Rick and recommend him and his clinic to anyone, but especially those with chronic challenging issues." **-Fiona B**

"What if you are planting a huge garden, but you don't have any tools? What if you are planning a long life, but you don't know the basics of movement, such as balance, strength, or stretching? Unfortunately, most of my life, I've spent clawing for answers to my pain, without any real tools. That just changed. I had been having back muscle problems for years when I began seeing Rick about two years ago. Rick diagnosed my muscle spasms immediately as a side bending issue and worked on my side muscles to correct it. He gave me a series of exercises which strengthened my trapezius muscles, my glutes, my hips, my sides, and my abs and showed me new ways to stand and move to prevent muscle spasms. I was pain-free for the first time in many years. When I again began experiencing severe muscle spasms the past year possibly as the result of a fall, I again saw Rick, who worked with me again to correct a new side bending problem and gave me more strength and balance exercises to prevent the muscle spasms. We discovered some of the positions in which I was playing the piano were contributing to muscle spasms. He encouraged me to work with my piano teacher to play in a healthy position which would not strain my back. In addition, he recommended the Alexander technique for healthy body skeletal and muscle movement and breathing and Pilates to further strengthen my core and balance. I am now pain-free again thanks to Rick's work with me, and am able to hike, ski, backpack, cycle, and play the piano in comfort. I am particularly grateful for the understanding he has given me about how my back, glutes, and abdominal muscles work together and the tools he has given me to keep my back strong and healthy for years to come. When my husband saw Rick for knee pain, he diagnosed it the minute he saw my husband walking toward him, and changed the way my husband was walking. My husband's pain was gone two days later, and he has been pain-free since. Rick provides each of his patients with handouts explaining the exercises he prescribes and illustrating how to do them. He also has a series of audios addressing proper body movements to prevent muscle pain and keep muscles strong. He has written several extremely informative books he calls *Fixing You*, which address neck, shoulder, and back pain, as well as knee and ankle pain. These books explain the origin of these pains, proper body movements, and provide exercises with illustrations to prevent pain and keep muscles strong." **-Ann N**

"As I stiffly approached Rick's system, I had little hope that my chronic back pain would ever be lessened. (In fact, I had accepted the very real possibility that I would just have to live with it.) Instead, I set out on a quad stretching adventure. Unlocking my knees and leaving a negative back habit behind loosened up muscles that had been causing my lower back pain. Twelve PT appointments brought me relief in my daily life activities, but especially in being able to pick up and carry my one-year-old granddaughter without immense discomfort. They worked my muscles hard, gave me excellent exercises to do at home, but provided me with a great forward progression to leave my back pain behind." **-K Wiedenfeld**

"I have had scoliosis since elementary school that I managed on my own while being active in sports. Once graduating and starting retail, my pain increased because I did not have good techniques to help the pain or to even stand the 'right' way. After working a labor-intensive retail job and going to school for a computer degree, my body began failing me, from dropping things to not being able to open my hands when I woke up. I did not go to the gym or walk anymore due to the pain all over my body. When I came here, I was very depressed and disappointed with where my young adult life was headed health-wise. Rick's system really helped me to open up and understand my body better. Why certain parts hurt or why I felt so twisted. The different stretches, workouts, and resting positions have helped me to work with my body to be in less pain and be able to manage the pain that will still come. I feel lighter physically and mentally. The book is also great." **-Katrina M**

"I started with lower-left-side back pain and left knee pain. Rick's system got me the exercises I need to perform to get my body aligned and my pain eliminated. Four visits were all it took." **-Jude K**

"The last 3-4 years, I was suffering severe pain around my upper rib cage area. I had a broken rib in the past, but my upper rib cage pain was much more severe. I took 1400-2100 mg ibuprofen, 500 mg Tylenol, and ibuprofen P.M. for the last three years. Sometimes I took 3000 mg ibuprofen a day, but I still had pain. Three weeks ago, my doctor sent me here. Rick Olderman found my trapezius muscle had zero function. I couldn't even move my shoulder blades. Then Rick gave me several exercises to recover that muscle and other exercises to strengthen the muscle. I learned postures were so important. For the last three weeks, I haven't had to take any pain pills. I am really happy now. I'm going back to the boxing gym. Thank you so much." **-Yutaka A**

"I first met Rick Olderman several years ago. My doctor sent me to him because I had been suffering with sciatica for several weeks, not sleeping, and unable to walk. My husband pushed my wheelchair into Rick's office. Rick smiled, looked into my eyes, and said, 'Nancy, we can fix this. This pain will soon be gone.' In one visit, Rick diagnosed the problem and sent me home with exercises to strengthen weak muscles and remain pain-free. I pushed my wheelchair out! I returned a few times to make sure I was healing. The sciatica never returned. I appreciate the quiet, gentle, caring, and professional courtesy of all Rick's staff. Over the years, I have returned several times for help with injuries or movement issues. Every time, Rick has been able to evaluate the problem and set me on the path of healing." **-Nancy G**

"I was originally referred for middle back pain, but also was having problems with hips. After several months of physical therapy and doing the recommended exercises, my back pain has improved considerably, and my hips bother me very little." **-Bob D**

"When I hobbled through the door, I had been unable to walk upright or sleep without pain for weeks. Learning how to move properly without harming myself from laziness was a challenge, but worth it! Everyone I worked with was very kind and efficient in getting me back into proper and mobile shape. It's funny but being excited just to be able to do house chores again is not something I expected, but I am enjoying!" **-Lisa B**

"I had really awful back pain. He spoke with confidence, knowledge, and encouragement and I followed his guidelines and now know how to keep healthy long-term. Thanks for all your help. It has been my pleasure. We are lucky you have such a passion." **-Peggy P**

"The *Back Pain* book helped me tremendously. My lower back pain is gone, I can walk up stairs, sleep, and sit with little pain. What I found different about this book from others:

1. Specific explanations of movement patterns that cause major back dysfunctions and pain. As much as we don't want to admit it and work on it, how we move affects muscles and bones and affects pain. Rick's explanations are very clear. I've read many articles/books that are either too dense and I don't understand it or I do a certain exercise without explaining what's being worked on. Rick explains things in a way I can understand and when I do the exercises, I know what I'm working on. My friends are amazed at my knowledge of muscles and movement now.
2. The best illustrations and explanations of how muscles work and are affecting the back pain that I have seen.
3. Specific exercises for specific back movement issues. Very clear exercises that also say what muscles are being worked and problems resolved. You can also get videos of the exercises that are great.
4. Suggestions on how to sit, stand, walk, and climb stairs. This helped me tremendously because as much as I don't want to work on my everyday movements, they are contributing, if not majorly causing, my problems.

"I love this whole series. This book contains super useful and easy-to-understand information. There are even helpful exercises to do that really helped my stiff low back area!" **-J Mulcahy**

SHOULDER

"I had a great experience working with Rick and his system. I hurt my shoulder playing tennis a while back and it was just never the same. Within a couple of weeks my range of motion was much better and then within two months I was back to playing tennis. I feel great and my shoulder feels better every day. Thank you."
-Chad P

"I was doing Pilates and felt something shift in my shoulder socket. One month later, an MRI confirmed another labral tear in the same shoulder in a different spot. The orthopedic surgeon could only suggest going back in to repair it again. I was HOPELESS!! How could this happen again? Why couldn't anyone help me figure out why this kept happening?

"The shoulder is definitely the most complex joint in the human body. Rick's book simplifies postural adjustments that will not only eliminate a great deal of pain but will make you aware of how much control you have over posture and pain. You can become aware of how you sit, stand, walk, and move and make it all more efficient to progress to more workouts with less pain! Hooray! What every injured person wants, right?

"Rick has helped me SO much with my shoulder pain! I owe all of the amazing changes I have made in my own movements to his simple principles. Rick's *Fixing You* series has inspired me to work on a new approach to teaching the Pilates method with a different postural model. My clients are responding beautifully and with such enthusiasm! The results have been amazing and it's only the beginning! Thank you, Rick, for SO much pain relief and professional inspiration!"
-Sarah Renee Weinberger, Pilates Partner, LLC

"When I started, my shoulder was extremely stiff due to 4+ months of no movement from a fracture. Stretching, isometrics, and finally strength-building gave me 100% use of my arm over 2–3 months of physical therapy. I feel whole again!" **-Jared W**

"I met Rick on February 6, 2010. Four months and three of his *Fixing You* books later, I can say I am a different person. I came to Rick with a pretty complex shoulder issue. I had torn my labrum (cartilage) in August 2008 and after 7 months and countless orthopedic/physical therapy opinions later, I was going under the knife. The surgery was a success and so was my 6 months of rehab. Did I mention I am a certified Pilates instructor?" **-Denver, CO**

"Though I'm not suffering too badly from shoulder issues, and I haven't done a whole lot of the exercises, this book doesn't skimp on explaining how shoulder blades (scapula), the collar bone, and a whole host of muscles work together. I ordered about seven books on shoulders and this one is great for combining a good overview of the various personally fixable problems and gives good advice and online videos to see the exercises." **-Thomas D**

"Rick Olderman's book series has improved my life considerably. As I go into my late 40s, my body is letting me know how much I abused it in my 20s and 30s as a drummer and a career bike messenger. Movement in my left shoulder has become a painful experience with something as simple as holding a basketball over my head. I had seriously started thinking this was something I just had to accept living with for the rest of my life. And, of course, this created a downward spiral because I was now gaining weight and exercising less because of the pain. I was browsing shoulder pain exercise books one day and I saw Rick Olderman's *Fixing You: Shoulder and Elbow Pain* and read some of the reviews. Every review I read was very positive and it excited me. When I started doing the exercises it really did feel like I was taking my first step towards repairing my left shoulder. I think the key to it is not just the exercises but understanding the mechanics of the shoulder and how it interacts with the rest of your body. I think this is the reason why this book series works so well. Before I read this, I'm not sure if I knew where my humerus was or my scapula, but Rick's easygoing explanations on how the body works makes this that much more enjoyable and approachable. Thanks, Rick, you've improved my quality of life." **-Robert C**

"If you are injured and searching for a quick fix, best of luck to you. But if you want to take charge of your healing, then by all means PUSH the button and order these ASAP! I began with *Fixing You: Neck Pain and Headaches* and had beyond incredible results. Then I went and ordered the ENTIRE series! No Joke. These books make sense, and the results are fantastic provided that you give the effort and work to do the exercises as stated. When I am done doing the exercises, I ice my neck and I feel normal. THIS is HUGE, when you've suffered pain from injuries. And to Dr. Olderman, if you read these, someday I'm going to personally shake your hand for giving me an escape route from surgery. I don't have the words to express my gratitude to you for the information found within the pages of your books. 'Thank you' seems so insufficient, but sincerely I Thank You!" **-Jennifer P**

"Rick and his team have been wonderful. They listen and always seem to get to the problem. Rick explains all the treatments and makes sure you are doing your exercises at home properly. My shoulder recovery has come along perfectly, and I know my recovery would not have been as successful without Rick's system."
-Ellen F

"Excellent book. The exercises provided immediate relief for my shoulder. When I looked at the exercises, I thought 'how could these exercises and stretches do anything?' Well, my shoulder feels much better, and I do the exercises/stretches regularly."
-Amazon Customer

"My shoulders and upper back had been getting progressively stiffer over the last 2–3 years. I had always been very flexible, so I found my restricted movements quite distressing. When the neck pain started and gave me occasional headaches, I saw some physical therapists and was given some exercises to do. It just made things worse, especially the headaches. I had

some massage therapy which helped for a bit, but the stiffness and pain returned as soon as I stopped. Then a few weeks ago, I read through this book and tried the exercises. They've certainly helped me. The stretches are very good, and the strengthening exercises have made some difference too. I'm back to the level of flexibility I had before, and my neck pain is so much better. And no headaches at all. I've still got a way to go to strengthen my upper back, but I now feel very motivated to do so."
-Amazon Customer

"I ended up getting the whole set. I love these books so, so much. It's easy to understand and it contains helpful exercises. Quick easy read full of super useful information. I can't recommend these books enough if you have a joint or some muscles that are acting up."
-J Mulcahy

"I have two very good physical therapists, but neither identified the underlying problem. Though my years of chronic pain are not gone, after weeks of work, I have the most improvement ever." **-Lori**

"I'm recovering from a dislocated shoulder, and I wanted to better educate myself to help me get through recovery and continue to strengthen and stretch to prevent a future injury." **-Amazon Customer**

"At first when I had just gotten the book, I was disappointed. I wanted to see a more detailed kind of book that would have more depth. But as soon as I started to read the book, I was hooked. The simplicity in which the material is described is just what I needed. And it turns out the information was right on spot! Needless to say, I fixed my shoulder problem due to the information that was given. This is a must for anyone with shoulder pain!"
-Amazon Customer

"I've gone for years with shoulder pain. I've seen doctors and I work out at the gym. But I didn't know where the pain came from until I read Rick's simple explanation, and it made total sense. Why can't the docs tell me that? Maybe they don't know or don't care? I emailed Rick and he got back to me in a matter of hours. I read his book and watched his online videos on how to properly do the exercises. $18 and a commitment to myself to do the simple, but highly effective exercises. I'm getting better and better every day." **-Amazon Customer**

"Thanks to this book, I now understand the mechanics of the shoulder blade interacting with the collarbone and shoulder joint, and Mr. Olderman's recommendations for movement have positively changed my biomechanics in everyday life. No more pain and discomfort!"
-M Benson

"This book really helped me learn how to hold my posture correctly to avoid the shoulder pain that I was experiencing. The exercises, done repeatedly, help ingrain proper posture. I highly recommend this quick read, with visuals, for anyone who would like to avoid surgery and still get rid of the pain!" **-Gracie M**

"I like the way the book is written. The author explains anatomy in just the right detail and the diagrams helped me especially to get the right muscles engaging. I think that's where I went wrong in the past with exercises ... always using the wrong muscles and making my pain worse. The website associated with the book is also very good and really helped me to perform the exercises properly. There are also some daily tips in the book, and I found these to be very useful too. It's a great little book and its size is part of its virtue. The exercises, once you master them, don't take too long either." **-Anna F**

"As a non-medical person, I found the book informative, easy to understand, and useful. It follows the same three-section format as the other books in the *Fixing You* series, which is helpful if you are familiar with any of them. The first section covers the nature of pain in general and is common to all the series (although heavily updated in the recently published *Fixing You: Back Pain*). It is essential reading as it provides a necessary foundation and link for all that follows. The second section covers the anatomy of the shoulder and elbow and is well described and illustrated. This part of the book also shows how pain, stiffness, etc. may occur in the area. It also gives a link to appropriate exercises listed in section three. This means you can go straight to your problem in section two and then directly to the exercise without reading the whole text—useful if pain strikes suddenly. The third section gives fully illustrated exercises to assist in overcoming pain referred to in section two. This section is excellent as the exercises are based on the author's experience of what works, and not simply copied from other texts. As you might have gathered, I have found great benefit in following the advice offered in this series of books, and very highly recommend them." **-Amazon Customer**

"I came to Rick's system after years of upper back pain and pelvic dysfunction. I have been through so many years of physical therapy, but I always had my back pain return. I have now incorporated all the postural changes Rick had given me and have been pain-free for three months already. The changes have been life-altering for me." **-Maureen W**

"Well, I must admit that I was skeptical at first. My pain is from Iliotibial Band Syndrome, and your videos did not address that specifically. But I persevered with the easy exercises and, once again, you are a genius! I slept last night with minimal pain. Thank you so very much. I will continue to walk the walk, study the exercises, and do them as well as I can (at age 72 years). I like these videos better than the older ones. Watching you work through them as you explain is most helpful. Also, the demonstration of alternative positions was just what I needed. While I'm exercising, I can hear your voice in my head telling me to go slowly. I need that!

"I think your techniques are life changing. When I first found your books on Amazon, I had been to doctors, physical therapists, physiatrists, chiropractors, etc. with no results. It seems they just don't know what they are doing. And I was spending hundreds of dollars! My back pain went away very quickly once I studied your techniques (and the McKenzie method, too) and it's been gone ever since.

MOTOR VEHICLE ACCIDENT

I have purchased 11 of your books, some to give away to other people in pain. But I wonder if they even read them. I know your method has to be studied and requires some perseverance and a learning curve, but it's so worth it! Sadly, I think most folks would rather have a shot, or a pill, or go under the surgical knife instead of working at fixing themselves. God bless you and give you success." **-Ruth**

"I was in a motorcycle accident. The doctor sent me to Rick's system to recover from injuries. They helped me with all the physical therapy that was needed to return to daily activity. They administered exercises and stretching to help get my gluteus maximus back to working properly. They answered all questions regarding the function of exercises and the whys." **-Sam P**

"When I first hobbled through the door in physical therapy, I could barely stand up straight. Turning my head, lifting my arm, basic everyday functions were difficult. Through treatment and attainable goal setting, I gradually became stronger and stronger. I am now well down the road to being physically my best self. I am a hair away from running a mile in 10 minutes (my personal best) and have lost almost all of the weight I gained since the accident. Rick and the rest of the staff are knowledgeable, great motivators, and just all-around awesome. I feel like I am twice the person I am than when I first walked through those doors." **-Terrence S**

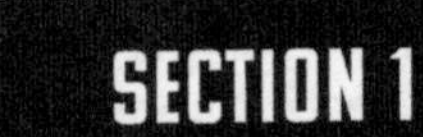

SECTION 1

THE UPPER BODY SYSTEM

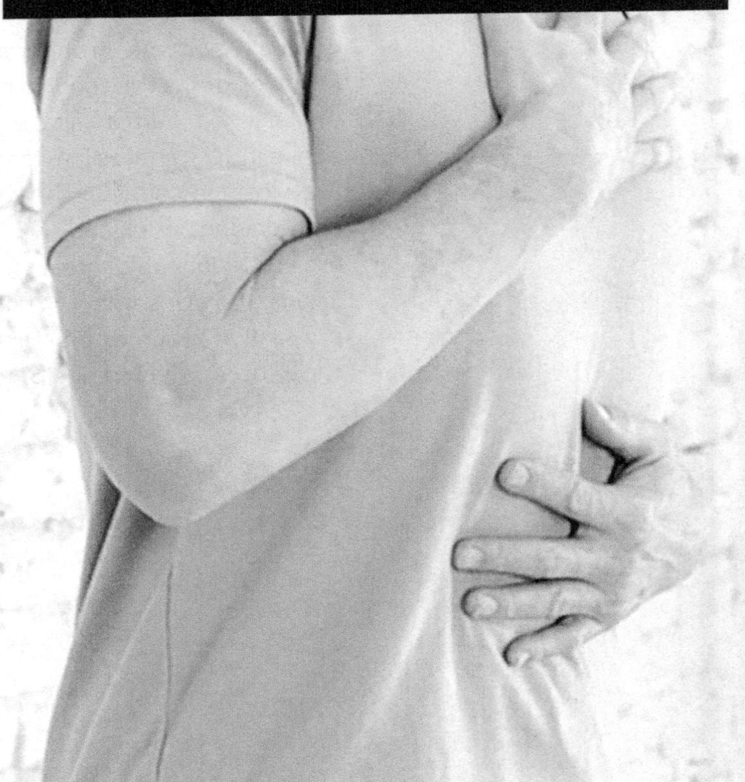

CHAPTER 3

How the Upper Body System Works

This chapter will lay the foundation for understanding what the upper body system is and how it works. You'll discover connections that previous treatment for your pain has either overlooked or not considered. To learn more about the muscles, bones, and biomechanics of this system, please read my books *Fixing You: Neck Pain & Headaches* and *Fixing You: Shoulder & Elbow Pain.*

You'll be surprised to learn that the upper body system is much simpler than you might imagine!

The information in this section will help you solve the following conditions:

- -Neck Pain/Headaches
- -Neck Hump (Dowager's Hump)
- -Shoulder Pain
- -Elbow Pain

Looking at a skeleton, you'll see that almost all of the bones are long and thin—like levers. There are two areas of the body, though, that have broad, flat bones: the pelvis and the shoulder blades.

Our skeletal system is primarily comprised of long bones, which can be thought of as levers. Broad, flat bones can be thought of as centers of function.

Most people intuitively understand that the pelvis is the center of function for the legs and low back (we'll get to that in Section 2, The Lower Body System). Similarly, the shoulder blades (scapulae) are the center of function for the arms, neck, and head, and thus house the culprits of, and solutions to, chronic upper body pain.

Once grasped, this basic idea shapes our understanding not only that the body works as a system, but also how it works as a system to both cause and solve pain.

The fact that the shoulder blade is the center of function for our upper body system might come as a surprise, especially given that no one has addressed your shoulder blades as the source of your pain before now. However, this is probably why you still wrestle with pain.

Numerous muscular and fascial attachments connect the shoulder blade to the neck and head. The shoulder blade and arm system weigh between 15 and 30 lbs. When the shoulder blades are not working well, stress is delivered to the neck and head via these connections. Because the neck bones and skull are the anchor points for these muscular attachments, they become tasked with holding up the weight of the shoulder girdle complex. The joints, discs, and ligaments in the neck and head respond to this constant stress by developing chronic pain, irritation, disc bulges, nerve root compression, etc.

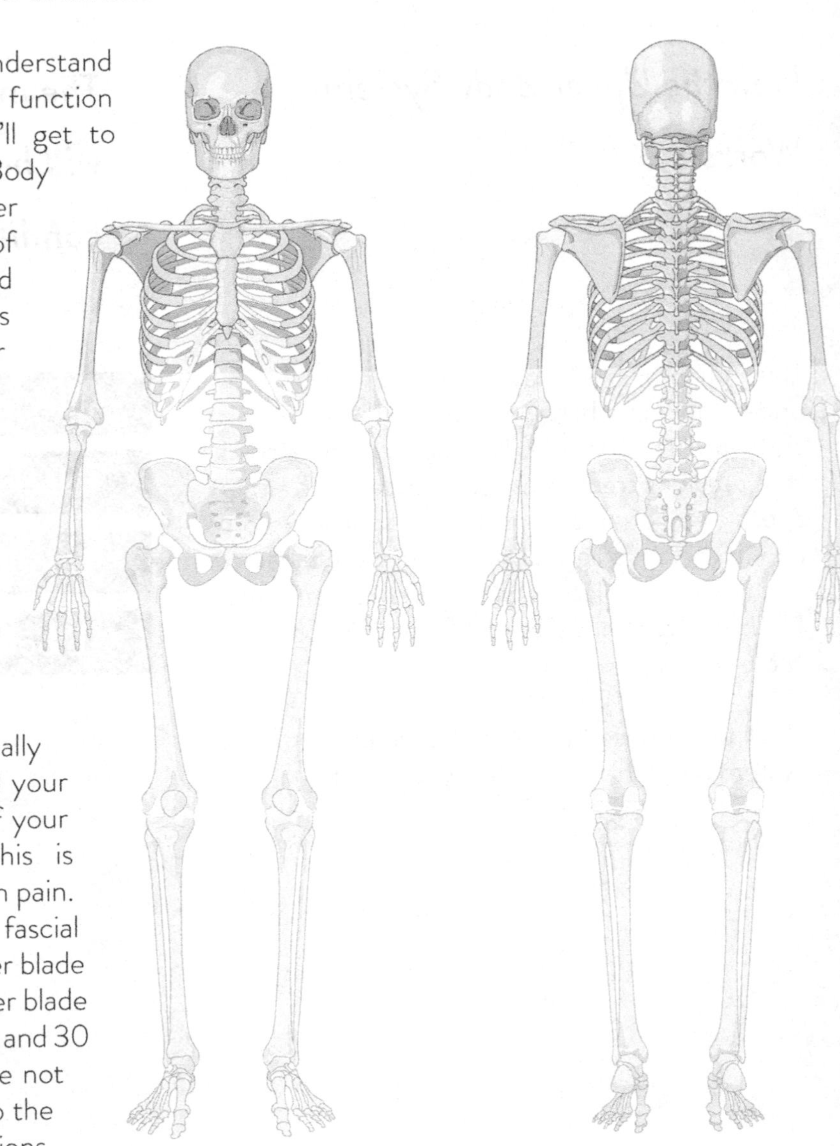

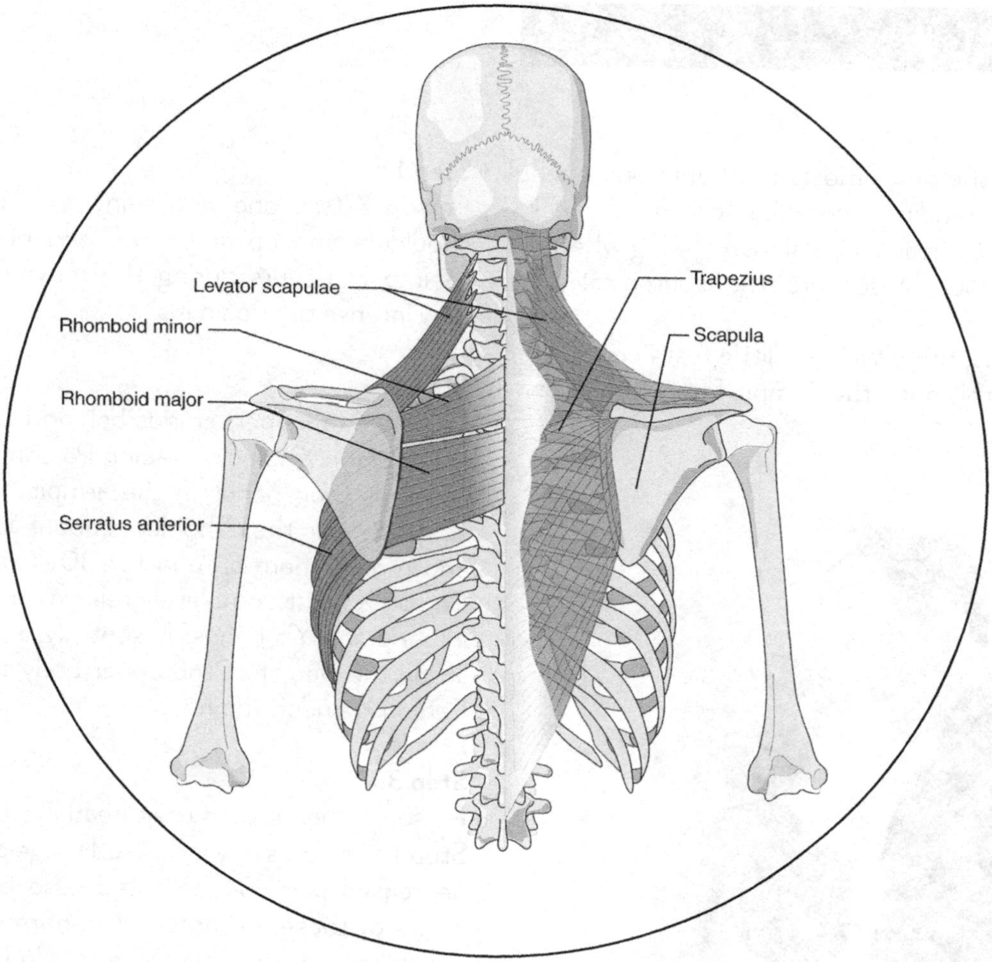

Numerous muscular attachments connect the shoulder blade to the neck bones and skull.

The shoulder blades operate under precise rules regarding how they should rest and move. More detail about what these rules are and how the muscular connections are involved can be found in my two books, *Fixing You: Neck Pain & Headaches* and *Fixing You: Shoulder & Elbow Pain*. We won't go into the rules here, but just know that when they are broken, pain results.

When viewing the upper body from a systems standpoint, it quickly becomes apparent that a pattern of problems that causes neck pain in one person can cause headaches in a second person and shoulder pain in a third. These problem patterns manifest as different types of pain in different people, due to genetics, exercise/sport history, older injuries, work history, diet, and emotional trauma or psychological stressors. This is why the same exercise recommended for neck pain will also work for headaches and shoulder pain, which simplifies solving pain.

Armpit Test

Probably the single most important component of understanding the root cause of neck, shoulder, or headache pain is knowing whether the shoulder blades are the source of the problem.

Luckily, there's a quick little test I created to figure this out—the Armpit Test. Here's how you do it.

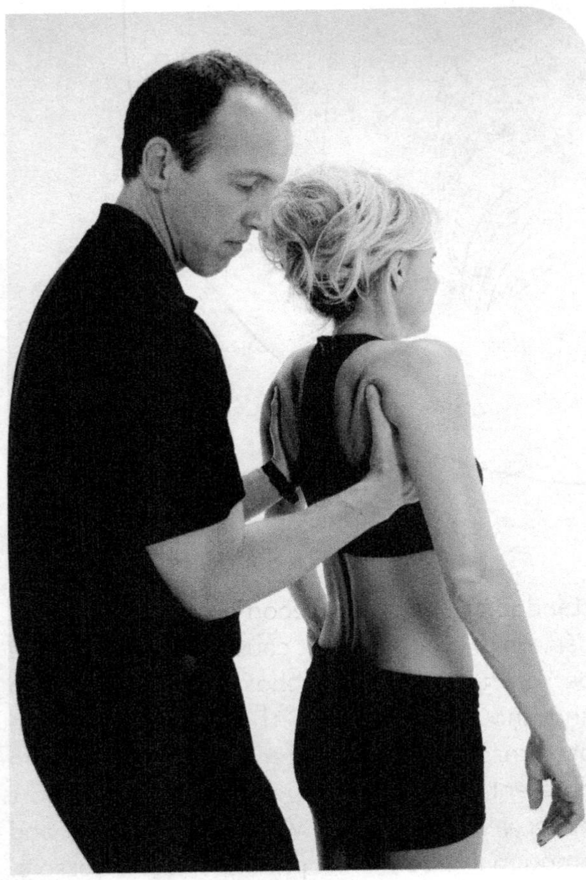

Lift the shoulders about 1/2–1 inch.

Step 1
Person X (the one with pain) looks over both shoulders and up and down and notes when their pain occurs during the movements and how intense their pain is.

Step 2
Person Y (a helper) stands behind Person X so that Person X's back is facing Person Y. Person Y places their hands in the armpits of Person X, gently lifts their shoulders about 1/2–1 inch, and moves them around for 30–60 seconds. Person X must completely relax their shoulders into Person Y's hands. Essentially, Person Y is lifting the weight of the upper body system off Person X's neck and head.

Step 3
Person X then moves their head like they did in Step 1 and notes any increased range of motion, decreased pain, or increased ease of motion. If any of these are noted, it confirms that the shoulder blades are playing a role in Person X's pain.

Step 4
Person Y gently lowers Person X's shoulders back down and removes their hands. Person X may notice that their pain increases again when moving their head. If the pain increases, the range of motion decreases, or the movement just doesn't feel quite as good, the shoulder blades are confirmed as the source of Person X's pain.

In my 25+ years as a physical therapist, I can't think of a single patient whose chronic neck, shoulder, or headache pain wasn't due to shoulder blade dysfunction. The one behavior that interferes with obtaining a clear result with this test is Person X being unable to fully relax their shoulders during the test. That is the case if they can't allow the weight of the shoulders to be unloaded from the neck and head during the 30–60 seconds required to complete this test. In this case, I recommend moving forward with this program anyway. The exercises are designed to fix this system and the pain will likely be solved.

Test/Retest to Find Your Gems

Just as important as understanding the source of the pain is knowing whether an exercise will actually help fix the problem. I've found that, when using systems-based solutions, pain reduces rapidly.

Test/retest is a powerful tool that I and my therapists have used in my clinic for years that will help you understand which exercises will be most helpful for you.

• • •

There are three steps required when using the test/retest tool.

Step 1

1 Perform a movement that consistently causes pain. For instance, with neck or shoulder pain, a painful movement might be turning your head side to side, as in the Armpit Test above, or moving your arm in a certain range. In my clinic, I ask patients to perform some activity that consistently triggers their pain and then note the range of motion, repetitions, or time it takes to experience the pain. Your solutions will be clearer if you drill down into these details. This is your test.

Step 2

2 Perform one of the recommended exercises from this book twice (two sets) using perfect form.

Step 3

3 Retest your painful movement or activity from Step 1 to see if you can perform the test with less pain, if you can perform more repetitions without pain, if you can perform the test for a longer period without pain, or if you just seem to have to search a little harder for your pain before finding it.

If you note an improvement, then this exercise is important in directly reducing your pain, and you should perform it with perfect form frequently throughout the day, to speed up your progress. Repeat this process for each exercise to home in on the exercises that will reduce your pain most quickly.

CLIENT CONNECTION

One day in my clinic, a man came to see me with an eight-year history of sciatic pain for which he'd been through two spinal surgeries and seen a multitude of practitioners. I asked him to perform an activity that caused his pain. I then gave him one exercise to perform for two sets. After completing the two sets, I asked him to perform the pain-causing movement again. He had no pain. In just a few seconds, we confirmed that the problem was not in his back but in his hip.

Eventually, you should be able to complete all exercises without pain. However, identifying the exercises that particularly decrease pain can be very helpful in getting you where you want to go a little faster.

Another benefit of understanding and solving pain from a systems point of view is that many of the exercises that solve, say, headaches will also solve shoulder pain, and vice versa. So, while these exercises fall under a single category, feel free to use them for other types of upper body pain.

Alright, let's get to the exercises!

CHAPTER 4

Neck Pain

"The author says that neck pain is generally caused by trouble with the shoulders. In other words, it radiates to another area. It's similar to how a bad hip can hurt in the groin. So, you won't find any neck exercises here. Not one. You'll find unique stretches and strengthening exercises for the shoulders. The good news is that your neck will stop hurting. At least mine has. No, it's not totally there yet. I've only used the book for three days. But my horrible neck pain is almost gone by doing these exercises. The 'neck' exercises in other books and on DVDs didn't work." **-Amazon Customer**

"Slightly different approach to neck pain. Glad somebody is writing this up. First book that described my symptoms exactly. Exercises are very simple and not time-consuming. When I do them it works." **-Amazon Customer**

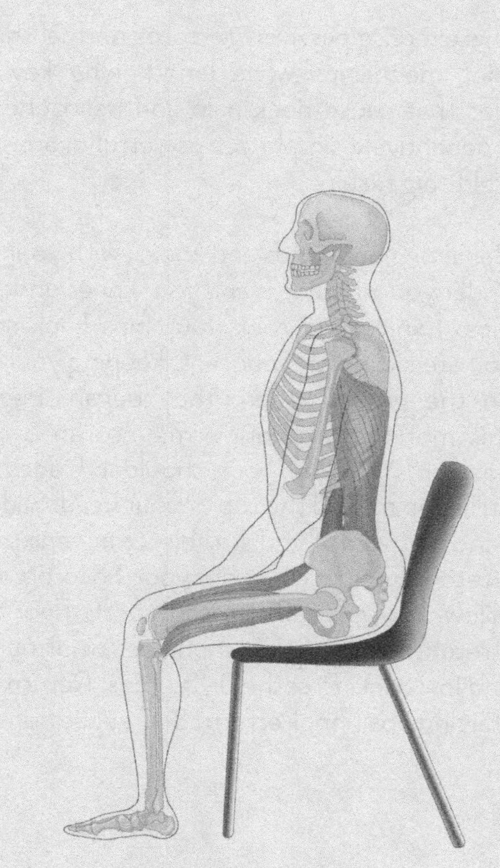

Neck pain is particularly responsive to treatment that fixes shoulder girdle dysfunction. This is because scapular muscles connect directly to the bones of the neck, thereby delivering stress to the spine.

All-Fours Rocking Stretch

This exercise passively restores normal shoulder joint mechanics while lengthening key muscles that cause neck pain and headaches. It is a deceptively simple yet powerful exercise that yields big results.

Begin on your hands and knees, with your hands under your shoulders and your knees under your hips. Exhale and rock your hips back so that you are sitting on your feet, keeping your hands on the ground where they began. Feel that this motion pulls your arms into an overhead position. Visualize your shoulder blades being pulled up toward the top of your head. Slide your hands forward, if you are able, to accentuate this stretch. Feel free to rest your head on a small pillow, if you prefer, for support. Feel a nice stretch through your shoulders or armpit area and low back. Breathe 3–5 times. Return to the starting position. Perform 3–5 repetitions.

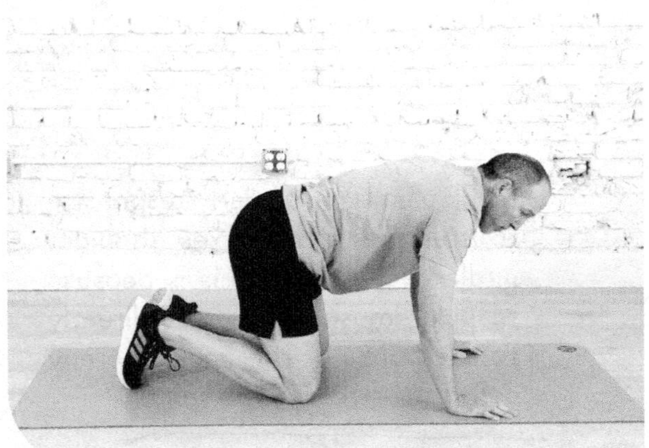

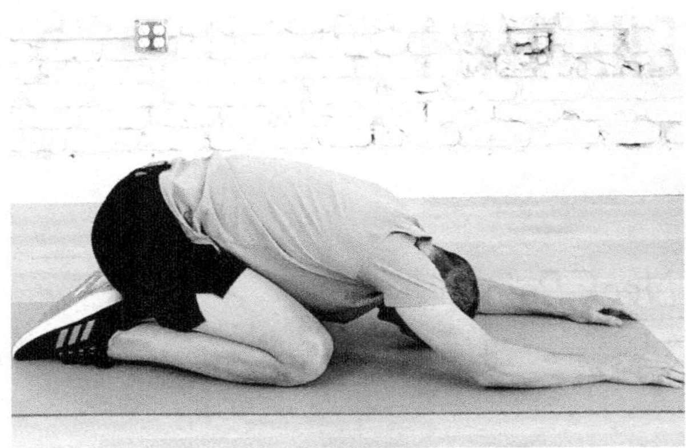

You should feel a stretch in your shoulders, chest, or arms during this exercise.

Take this stretch up a notch after sitting back on your heels by walking both hands to the left. Take three breaths and then walk your hands to the right. If your neck, shoulder, or headache pain is on one side, for example the right side, you'll likely find that your right shoulder and rib cage feel tighter. Solving that tightness will help solve your pain.

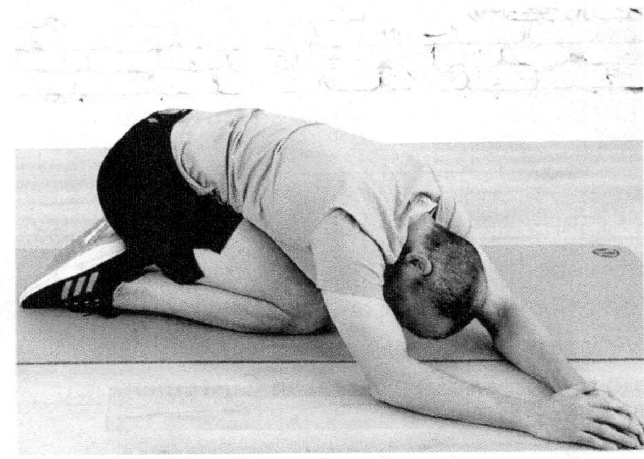

Sidebending while stretching can help you solve unilateral tightness contributing to your pain.

Arm Slides on the Wall

This exercise improves shoulder girdle movement and strengthens the key muscles involved in elevating the shoulder blades.

Begin with your right hand. Stand a few inches from the wall. Place your elbow and the pinky side of your hand on the wall. Make sure that your elbow is slightly below the level of your shoulder.

Slowly slide your hand up the wall. When your elbow is level with your shoulder, shrug your shoulder up to assist in elevating your shoulder blade. Continue gradually shrugging your shoulder as your arm slides up. Feel how elevating your shoulder blade pushes your hand further up the wall.

Stop before you feel any pain. If there is no pain, reach as high as you can and lean into the wall to accentuate the lengthening of your right rib cage and the elevation of your shoulder blade. Hold for three breaths.

Slide your arm down, allowing your shoulder blade to linger in that elevated position for just a second or two. Then feel your shoulder blade and arm return to the starting position together. Perform 5–10 repetitions. This should be pain-free, and your arm should be able to fully slide up the wall with an elevated scapula. Repeat on the other side.

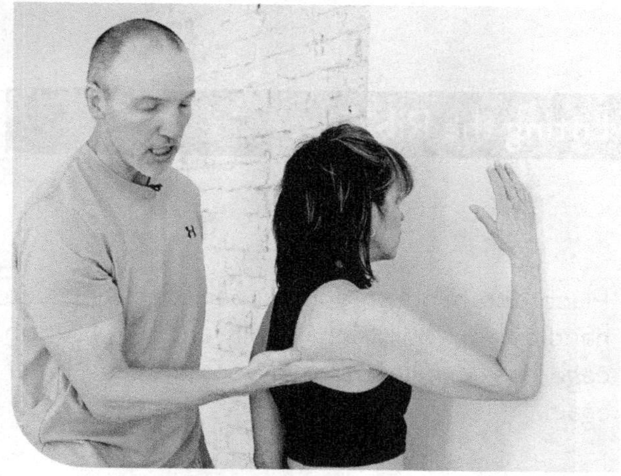

Begin with the pinky side of your hand on the wall and your elbow below shoulder height.

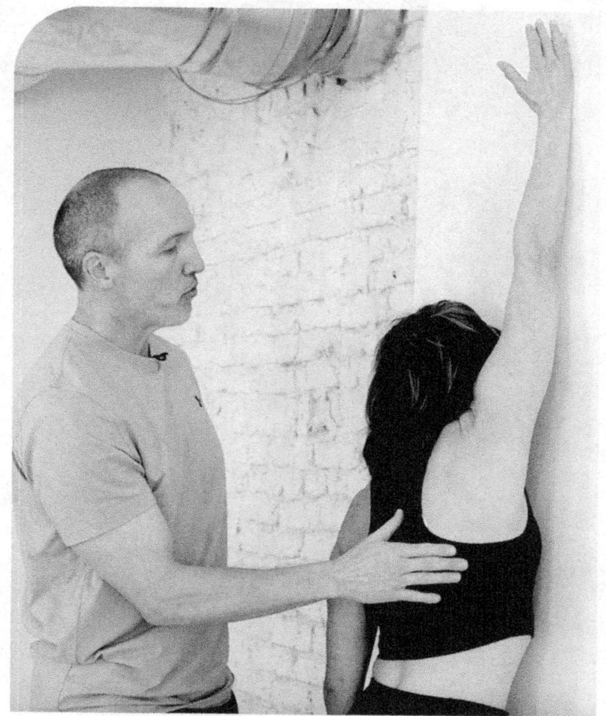

Finish by reaching as high as you can without pain.

Lifting the Rib Cage

Place one hand on your upper chest and one hand on your belly. Inhale fully and feel your rib cage rise. Exhale and feel your rib cage lower again.

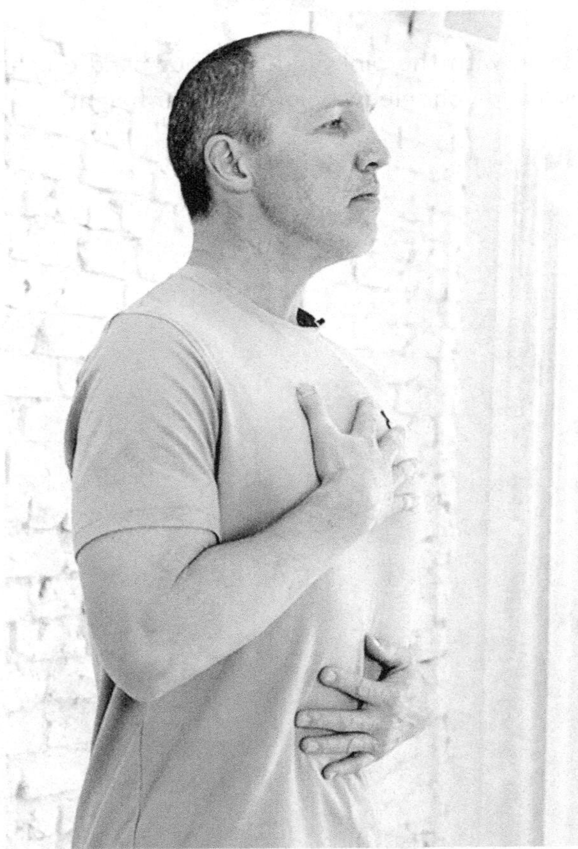

Gently lift your rib cage while relaxing your arms to create a better posture strategy.

Inhale again, feeling your rib cage rise, and allow it to fall again upon exhalation, but not quite all the way. Allow it to remain about 1–2 millimeters higher than normal. Feel free to exhale completely.

Notice that your stomach muscles have just turned on very slightly, without your conscious awareness. These core muscles naturally engage to support the trunk and upper body when posture is correct, holding the rib cage slightly higher than usual. This gentle contraction is all that is necessary to hold up the trunk. Notice that it requires no effort or active contraction of the stomach muscles on your part.

Now, allow your arms to rest by your sides. Roll your shoulders around to completely relax them. They should feel like two loose and dangling ropes hanging by your sides. Notice that when you've completely relaxed your arms, your stomach muscles have also turned off. This is because faulty posture strategies can cause shoulder muscle contraction rather than natural core activation. This is not what the shoulder system is designed to do. This is one of the patterns of stressors contributing to most upper body system chronic pain conditions. Practice creating improved posture this way by learning to remove your arms from the equation.

Fix Pain-Causing Habits

Upper Body Ergonomics

How you use your body can contribute to the development of the tight or weak muscles that are targeted in this program. Ergonomics plays a significant role in upper body pain. Follow this recommendation to adapt your workstation to reduce the stress on your upper body system.

When sitting at your workstation, your upper arms should be resting at your sides, about where the seam of your shirt is, and lightly touching your trunk. Particularly if the Armpit Test caused pain relief when your shoulder blades were lifted, the arms of your chair should be positioned at a height that causes your shoulders to be lifted 1/2–1 inch higher than normal.

With your upper arms in this position, wherever your hands are is where your keyboard should be. Any reaching or shifting from this position causes the shoulder and neck muscles to activate and strain.

Most chair arms, however, do not adjust enough to support this position. If this is the case with your chair, fold a bed pillow in half and stuff it between your forearm and the arm of the chair on both sides. This will create a broader, higher, and more comfortable platform on which to rest your upper body system while you work.

Make this change for the next week and notice your neck, shoulder, or headache pain diminish.

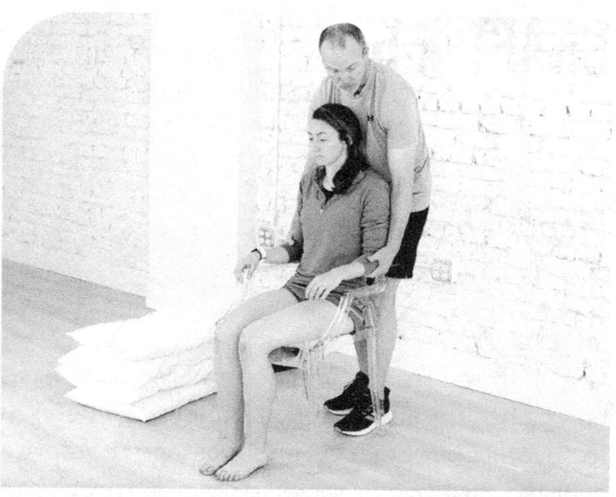

When sitting, your upper arms should rest at your sides.

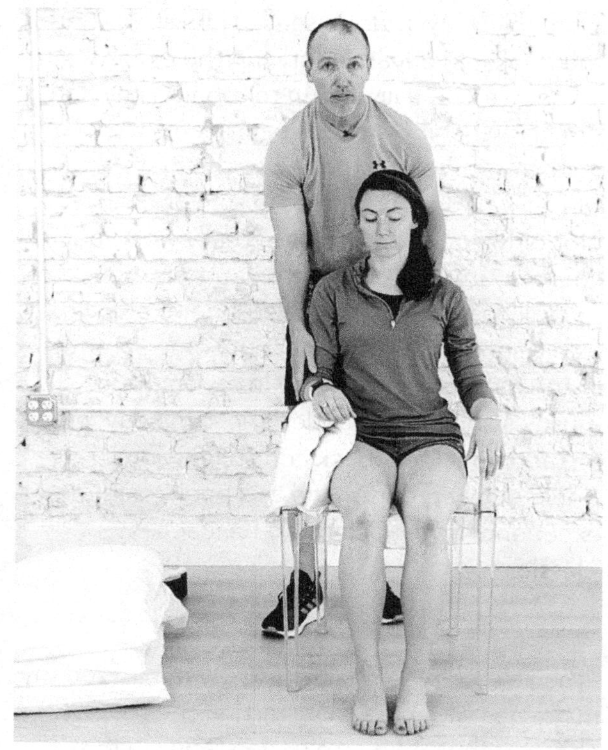

Use a pillow to help achieve an ideal platform for your arms.

CHAPTER 5

Headaches

"I've suffered from migraines and tension headaches for about ten years now. I've been to several chiropractors and massage therapists over the past five or six years, but the problem never completely went away. Nobody ever mentioned that the root of the problem could be in my shoulders, but after reading the book it completely made sense. So, I finished reading the book and began practicing the exercises in it as well as really trying to monitor my bad slouching habit. My neck pain seems to have gone away already. Today was the first day in a while that I did not get some sort of headache. Not only do the exercises actually work, but I'm really impressed with the author. He seems to really care and wants everyone to be pain-free. I sent him an email about some soreness that I started experiencing in my trapezius muscles and he responded the same day, giving me additional feedback and suggestions. I would highly recommend this book to anyone experiencing neck pain and headaches."
-Jessica

"The stretching exercises greatly minimized my migraines within days of starting the routine. The book helped me to understand what was going on." **-Don**

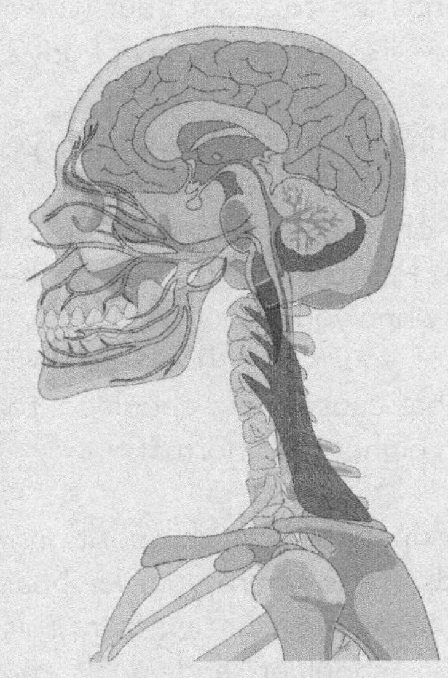

Solving shoulder girdle issues is an extremely effective way to eliminate chronic or recurring headaches. This strategy has been successful for tension or migraine headaches and has even been effective for a few cases of trigeminal neuralgia.

All-Fours Rocking Stretch

This exercise passively restores normal shoulder joint mechanics while lengthening key muscles that cause neck pain and headaches. It is a deceptively simple yet powerful exercise that yields big results.

Begin on your hands and knees with your hands under your shoulders and your knees under your hips. Exhale and rock your hips back so that you are sitting on your feet, keeping your hands on the ground where they began. Feel that this motion pulls your arms into an overhead position. Visualize your shoulder blades being pulled up toward the top of your head. Slide your hands forward, if you are able, to accentuate this stretch. Feel free to rest your head on a small pillow, if you prefer, for support. Feel a nice stretch through your shoulders or armpit area and low back. Breathe 3–5 times. Return to the starting position. Perform 3–5 repetitions.

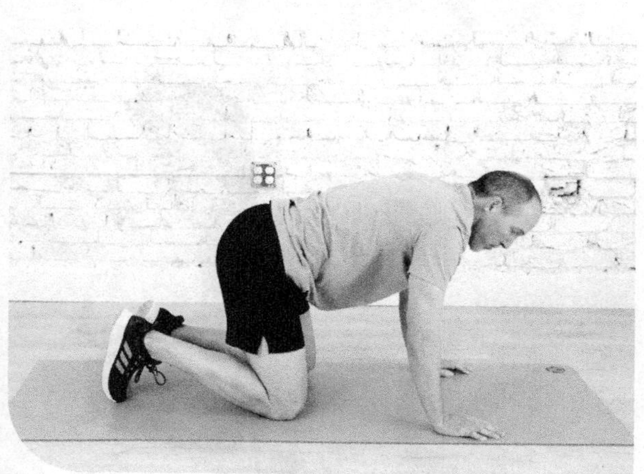

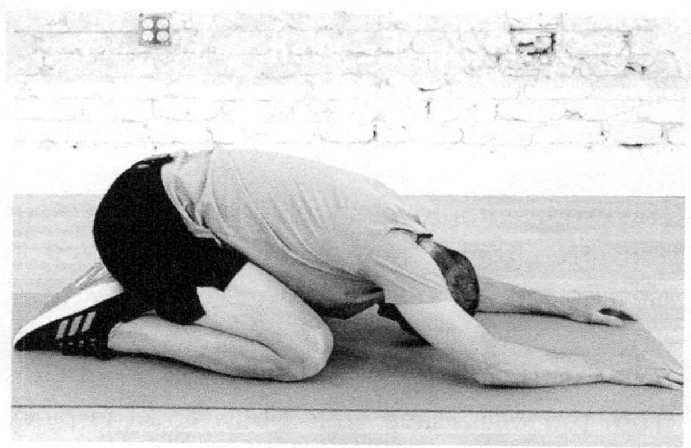

You should feel a stretch in your shoulders, chest, or arms during this exercise.

Take this stretch up a notch after sitting back on your heels by walking both hands to the left. Take three breaths and then walk your hands to the right. If your neck, shoulder, or headache pain is on one side, for example the right side, you'll likely find that your right shoulder and rib cage feel tighter. Solving that tightness will help solve your pain.

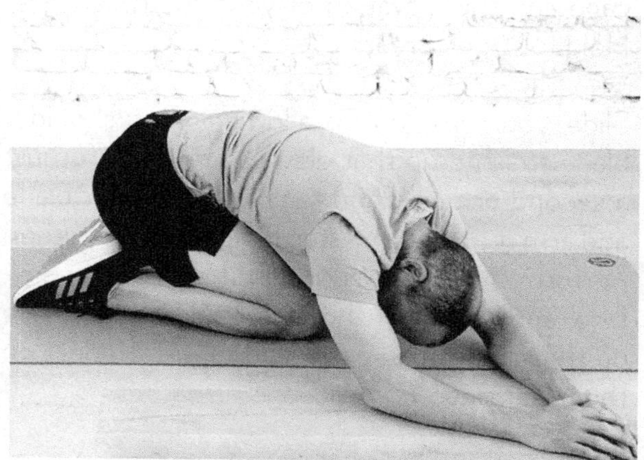

Sidebending while stretching can help you solve unilateral tightness contributing to your pain.

Arm Slides on the Wall

This exercise improves shoulder girdle movement and strengthens the key muscles involved in elevating the shoulder blades.

Begin with your right hand. Stand a few inches from the wall. Place your elbow and the pinky side of your hand on the wall. Make sure that your elbow is slightly below the level of your shoulder.

Slowly slide your hand up the wall. When your elbow is level with your shoulder, shrug your shoulder up to assist in elevating your shoulder blade. Continue gradually shrugging your shoulder as your arm slides up. Feel how elevating your shoulder blade pushes your hand further up the wall.

Stop before you feel any pain. If there is no pain, reach as high as you can and lean into the wall to accentuate the lengthening of your right rib cage and the elevation of your shoulder blade. Hold for three breaths.

Slide your arm down, allowing your shoulder blade to linger in that elevated position for just a second or two. Then feel your shoulder blade and arm return to the starting position together. Perform 5–10 repetitions. This should be pain-free, and your arm should be able to fully slide up the wall with an elevated scapula. Repeat on the other side.

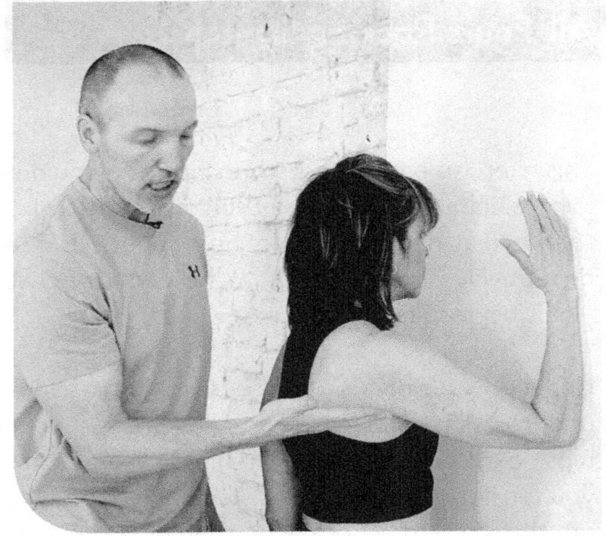

Begin with the pinky side of your hand on the wall and your elbow below shoulder height.

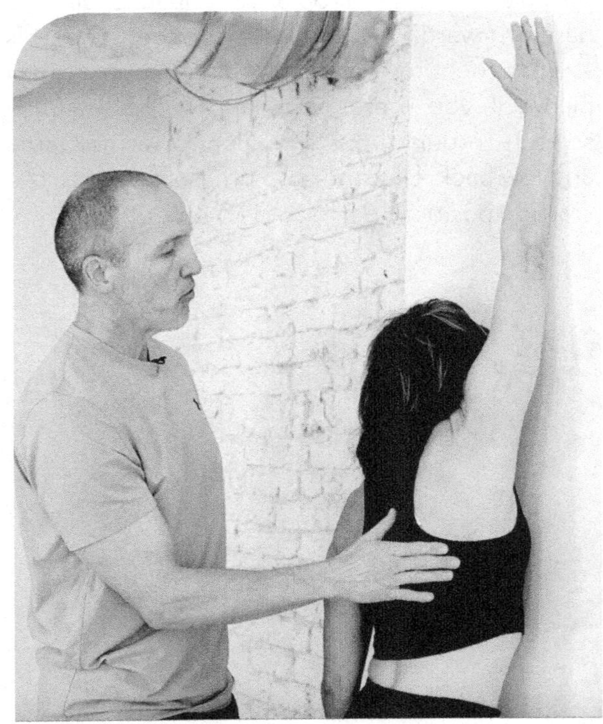

Finish by reaching as high as you can without pain.

Lifting the Rib Cage

Place one hand on your upper chest and one hand on your belly. Inhale fully and feel your rib cage rise. Exhale and feel your rib cage lower again.

Inhale again, feeling your rib cage rise, and allow it to fall again on the exhale, but not quite all the way. Allow it to remain about 1–2 millimeters higher than normal. Feel free to exhale completely.

Notice that your stomach muscles have just turned on very slightly without your conscious awareness. These core muscles naturally engage to support the trunk and upper body when posture is correct, holding the rib cage slightly higher than usual. This gentle contraction is all that is necessary to hold up the trunk. Notice that it requires no effort or active contraction of the stomach muscles on your part.

Now, allow your arms to rest by your sides. Roll your shoulders around to completely relax them. They should feel like two loose and dangling ropes hanging by your sides. Notice that, when you've completely relaxed your arms, your stomach muscles have also turned off. This is because faulty posture strategies can cause shoulder muscle contraction rather than natural core activation. This is not what the shoulder system is designed to do. This is one of the patterns of stressors contributing to most upper body system chronic pain conditions. Practice creating improved posture this way by learning to remove your arms from the equation.

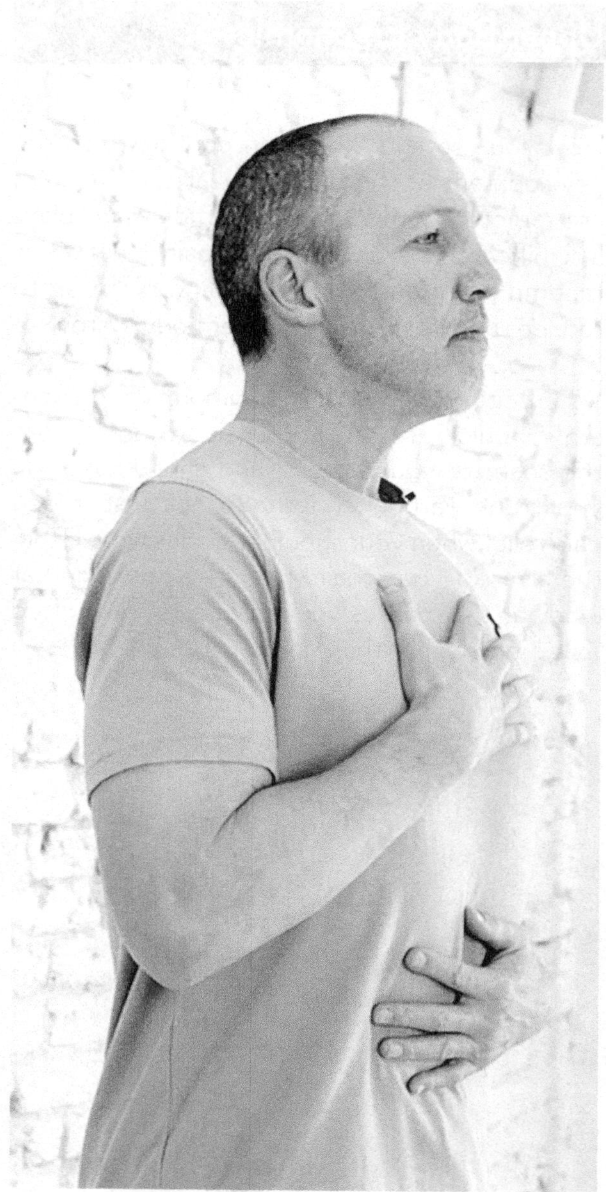

Gently lift your rib cage while relaxing your arms to create a better posture strategy.

Fix Pain-Causing Habits

Upper Body Ergonomics

How you use your body can contribute to the development of the tight or weak muscles that are targeted in this program. Ergonomics plays a significant role in upper body pain. Follow this recommendation to adapt your workstation to reduce the stress on your upper body system.

When sitting at your workstation, your upper arms should be resting at your sides, about where the seam of your shirt is, and lightly touching your trunk. Particularly if the Armpit Test caused pain relief when your shoulder blades were lifted, the arms of your chair should be positioned at a height that causes your shoulders to be lifted 1/2–1 inch higher than normal.

With your upper arms in this position, wherever your hands are is where your keyboard should be. Any reaching or shifting from this position causes the shoulder and neck muscles to activate and strain.

Most chair arms, however, do not adjust enough to support this position. If this is the case with your chair, fold a bed pillow in half and stuff it between your forearm and the arm of the chair on both sides. This will create a broader, higher, and more comfortable platform on which to rest your upper body system while you work.

Make this change for the next week and notice your neck, shoulder, or headache pain diminish.

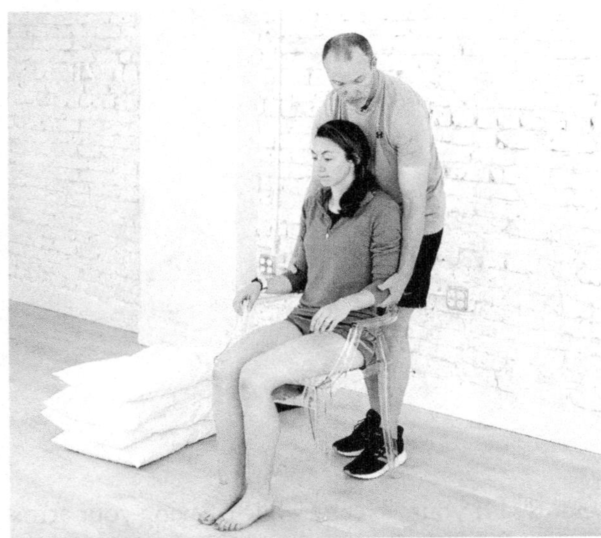

When sitting, your upper arms should rest at your sides.

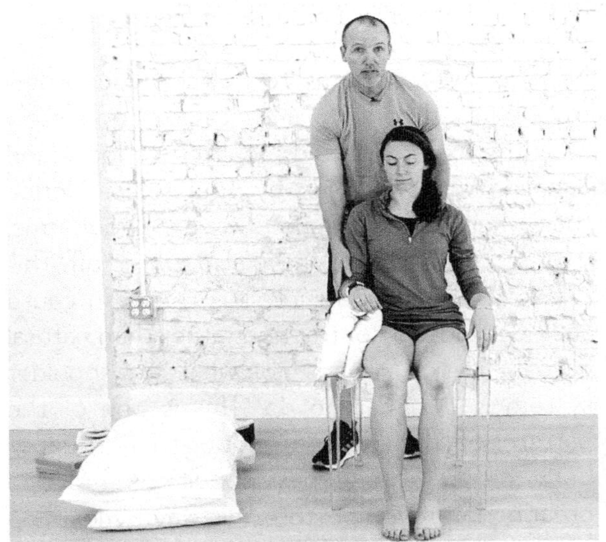

Use a pillow to help achieve an ideal platform for your arms.

CHAPTER 6

Neck Hump (Dowager's Hump)

"Here I was, bravely picking up one more book for chronic neck and shoulder pain, when I think I have tried, done, and read every possible approach (for many years, no relief, or worse, an exacerbation of pain). The very simple, clear, and subtle adjustments proposed by Rick Olderman have immediately given me a measure of relief and a huge feeling of hope. The exercises and conscious re-positioning are so logical and gentle that they also calm all the despairing thoughts that often accompany pain." **-Amazon Customer**

"It is a very good book that includes a lot of good stretches and anatomical reasons for neck pain. I recommend it highly." **-Joy O**

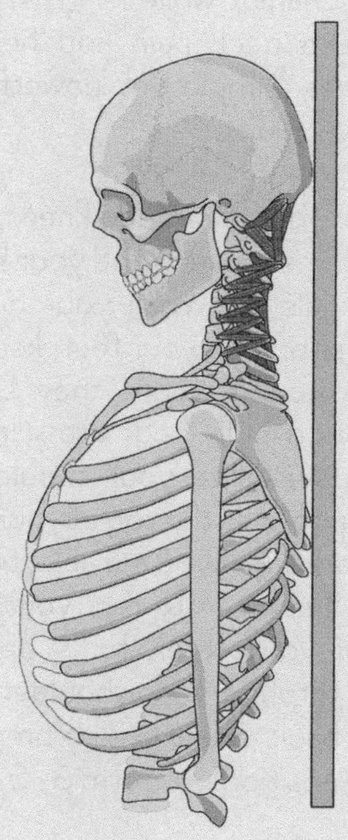

Neck humps occur at the transition between the curve of the neck and the curve of the midback. I have included a video online showing a case in which a neck hump was instantly eliminated simply by adopting a correct posture strategy.

All-Fours Rocking Stretch

This exercise passively restores normal shoulder joint mechanics while lengthening key muscles that cause neck pain and headaches. It is a deceptively simple yet powerful exercise that yields big results.

Begin on your hands and knees, with your hands under your shoulders and your knees under your hips. Exhale and rock your hips back so that you are sitting on your feet, keeping your hands on the ground where they began. Feel that this motion pulls your arms into an overhead position. Visualize your shoulder blades being pulled up toward the top of your head. Slide your hands forward, if you are able, to accentuate this stretch. Feel free to rest your head on a small pillow, if you prefer, for support. Feel a nice stretch through your shoulders or armpit area and low back. Breathe 3–5 times. Return to the starting position. Perform 3–5 repetitions.

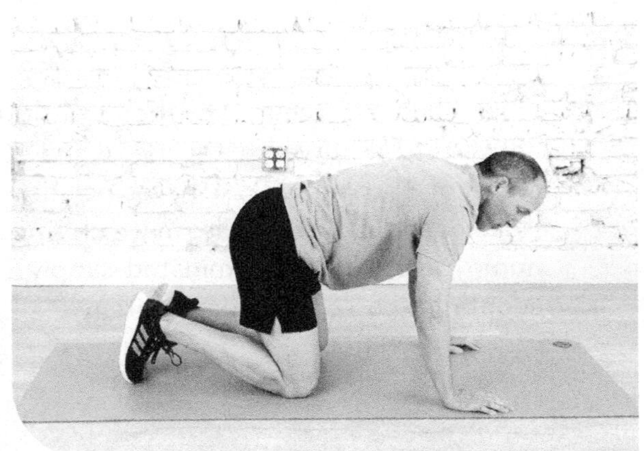

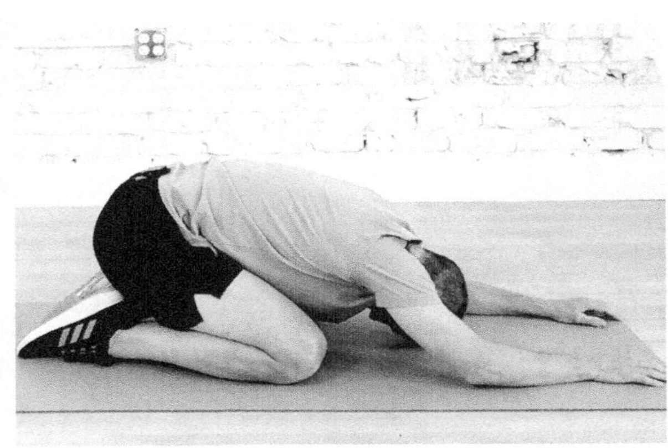

You should feel a stretch in your shoulders, chest, or arms during this exercise.

Take this stretch up a notch after sitting back on your heels by walking both hands to the left. Take three breaths and then walk your hands to the right. If your neck, shoulder, or headache pain is on one side, for example the right side, you'll likely find that your right shoulder and rib cage feel tighter. Solving that tightness will help solve your pain.

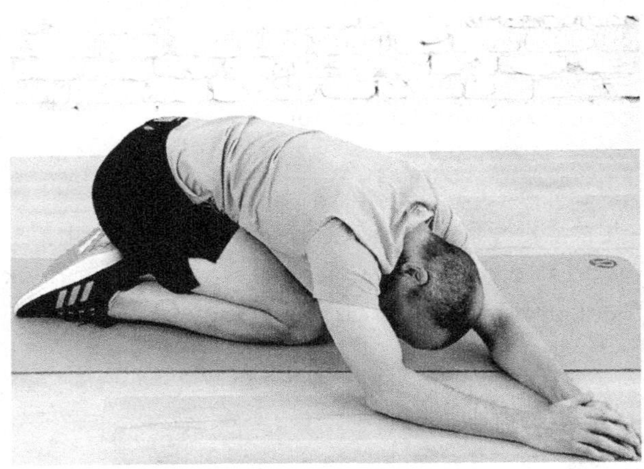

Sidebending while stretching can help you solve unilateral tightness contributing to your pain.

Arm Slides on the Wall

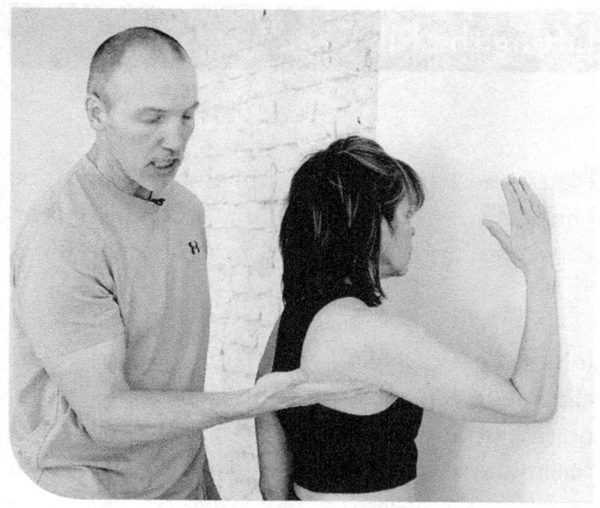
Begin with the pinky side of your hand on the wall and your elbow below shoulder height.

This exercise improves shoulder girdle movement and strengthens the key muscles involved in elevating the shoulder blades.

Begin with your right hand. Stand a few inches from the wall. Place your elbow and the pinky side of your hand on the wall. Make sure that your elbow is slightly below the level of your shoulder.

Slowly slide your hand up the wall. When your elbow is level with your shoulder, shrug your shoulder up to assist in elevating your shoulder blade. Continue gradually shrugging your shoulder as your arm slides up. Feel how elevating your shoulder blade pushes your hand further up the wall.

Stop before you feel any pain. If there is no pain, reach as high as you can and lean into the wall to accentuate the lengthening of your right rib cage and the elevation of your shoulder blade. Hold for three breaths.

Slide your arm down, allowing your shoulder blade to linger in that elevated position for just a second or two. Then feel your shoulder blade and arm return to the starting position together. Perform 5–10 repetitions. This should be pain-free, and your arm should be able to fully slide up the wall with an elevated scapula. Repeat on the other side.

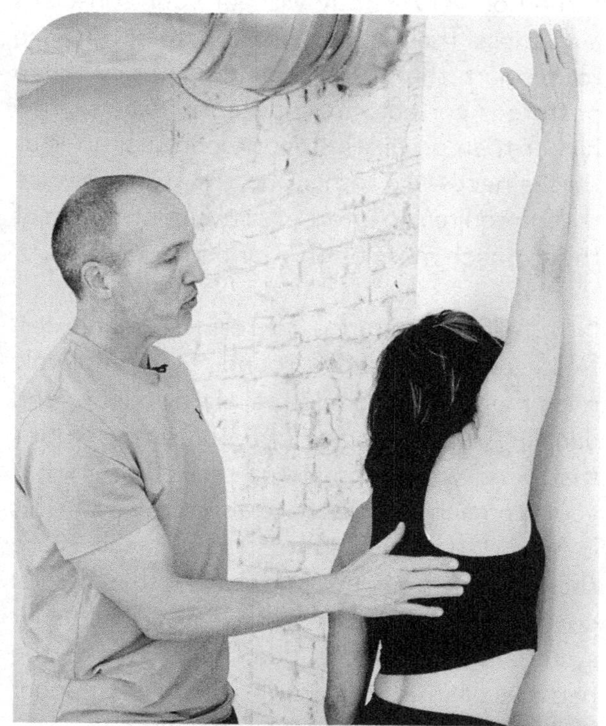
Finish by reaching as high as you can without pain.

Lifting the Rib Cage

Place one hand on your upper chest and one hand on your belly. Inhale fully and feel your rib cage rise. Exhale and feel your rib cage lower again.

Inhale again, feeling your rib cage rise, and allow it to fall again on the exhalation, but not quite all the way. Allow it to remain about 1–2 millimeters higher than normal. Feel free to exhale completely.

Notice that your stomach muscles have just turned on very slightly without your conscious awareness. These core muscles naturally engage to support the trunk and upper body when posture is correct, holding the rib cage slightly higher than usual. This gentle contraction is all that is necessary to hold up the trunk. Notice that it requires no effort or active contraction of the stomach muscles on your part.

Now, allow your arms to rest by your sides. Roll your shoulders around to completely relax them. They should feel like two loose and dangling ropes hanging by your sides. Notice that, when you've completely relaxed your arms, your stomach muscles have also turned off. This is because faulty posture strategies can cause shoulder muscle contraction rather than natural core activation. This is not what the shoulder system is designed to do. This is one of the patterns of stressors contributing to most upper body system chronic pain conditions.

Practice creating improved posture this way by learning to remove your arms from the equation.

Note: Please see my video clip of someone eliminating their neck hump in about 30 seconds by simply using these principles.

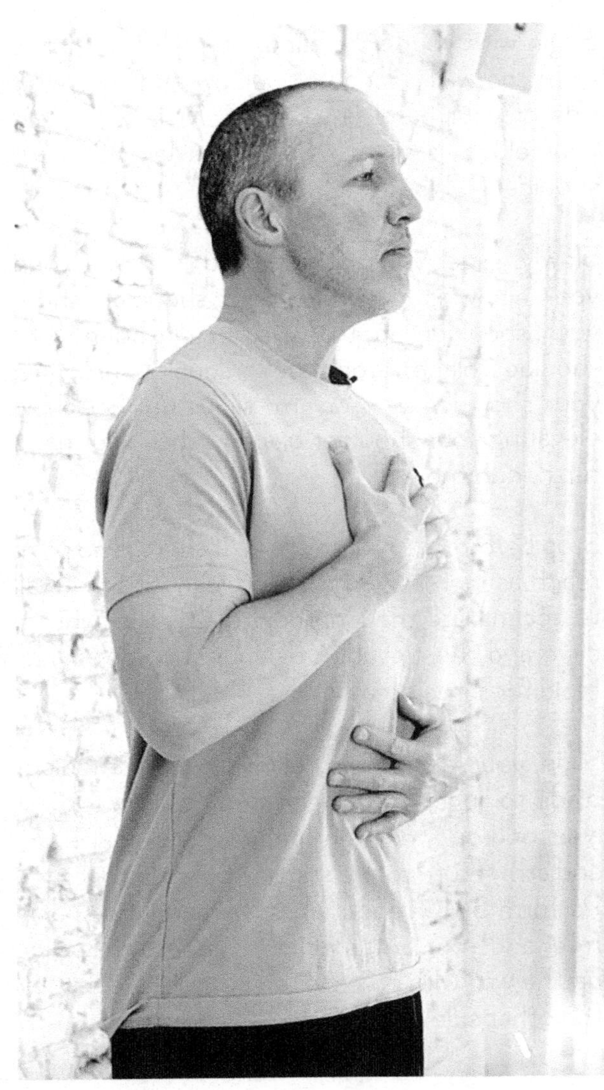

Gently lift your rib cage while relaxing your arms to create a better posture strategy.

Fix Pain-Causing Habits

Upper Body Ergonomics

How you use your body can contribute to the development of the tight or weak muscles that are targeted in this program. Ergonomics plays a significant role in upper body pain. Follow this recommendation to adapt your workstation to reduce the stress on your upper body system.

When sitting at your workstation, your upper arms should be resting at your sides, about where the seam of your shirt is, and lightly touching your trunk. Particularly if the Armpit Test caused pain relief when your shoulder blades were lifted, the arms of your chair should be positioned at a height that causes your shoulders to be lifted 1/2–1 inch higher than normal.

With your upper arms in this position, wherever your hands are is where your keyboard should be. Any reaching or shifting from this position causes the shoulder and neck muscles to activate and strain.

Most chair arms, however, do not adjust enough to support this position. If this is the case with your chair, fold a bed pillow in half and stuff it between your forearm and the arm of the chair on both sides. This will create a broader, higher, and more comfortable platform on which to rest your upper body system while you work.

Make this change for the next week and notice your neck, shoulder, or headache pain diminish.

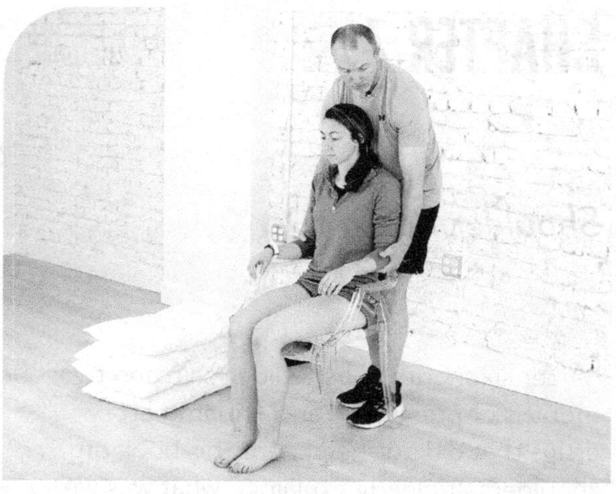

When sitting, your upper arms should rest at your sides.

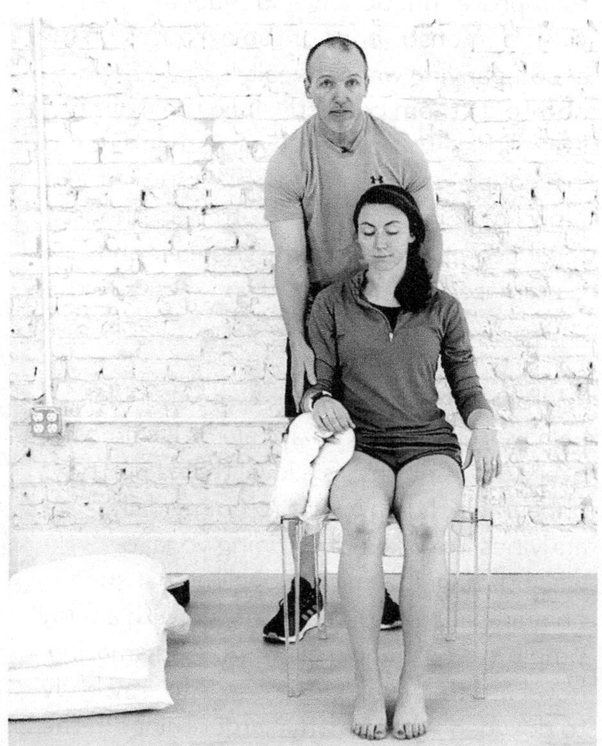

Use a pillow to help achieve an ideal platform for your arms.

CHAPTER 7

Shoulder Pain

"After six months of shoulder pain and two months of prescribed anti-inflammatory drugs that did not help, I got this book on shoulders. It clearly explained what was wrong in terms of how muscles, tendons, and joints all work together, and it gave exercises to do to improve functioning and reduce pain. The video demonstrations of the exercises on the accompanying website really helped explain how to do them correctly. I did the exercises just a little—three times every other day—and in a couple of weeks I felt 85% improvement. Now I'm doing them more often and hoping to regain complete use of my shoulder and arm. I was amazed." **-J Todd**

"Before coming to see Rick, my shoulder pain was easily an 8 on a scale of 10 almost every day. And that is a level that is pretty unbearable. I didn't want to do my daily activities like bike riding, doing yoga, or weightlifting. It is mind-boggling that such unbearable pain can be managed with a fairly simple strengthening exercise. And amazing how hard that simple exercise is for my body to do when I do so many harder things in the gym. Just shows how much I need it! Rick is incredibly helpful, and I know he can help me every time—he is the only one I've been to that can fix this for me." **-Jaymie H**

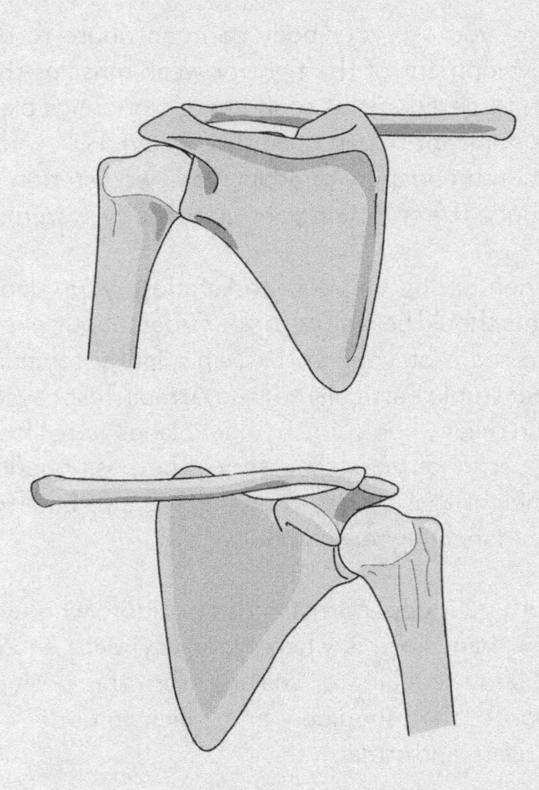

While the exercises described in Chapters 4-6 do address shoulder pain, the following exercises are more specific to the shoulder joint. Because we are solving problems in the upper body system, these shoulder exercises are also appropriate for treating neck and headache pain and fixing a neck hump.

Mid-Trapezius Strengthening

Because this exercise requires an awareness of how your shoulder blade is moving, it's best if someone can observe you, to help correct any errors in the movement. Alternatively, you can take a video of yourself to observe and correct any errors.

Master each level of this exercise before moving on to the next level.

Level 1. Lie on your stomach with your arms by your sides and your palms facing the ceiling. If this position is uncomfortable for your back or neck, place a bed pillow under your trunk. Feel free to rest your forehead on the arm you are not exercising if this is more comfortable.

Beginning with your stronger side, squeeze your shoulder blade so that it moves directly toward your spine—not down toward your hips or up toward your head—keeping your hand resting on the ground.

Hold for three breaths, noting how successful or easy this is.

Repeat three times. Switch to the other side.

Level 2. Perform Level 1. With your shoulder blade squeezed toward your spine, lift your palm a quarter of an inch off the ground. Maintain the correct shoulder blade position while holding your hand off the ground, with your palm facing the ceiling and knuckles facing the ground.

Hold for three breaths, noting how successful or easy this is. Lower your entire arm and shoulder blade together as one unit back to the ground to rest.

Repeat three times. Switch to the other side.

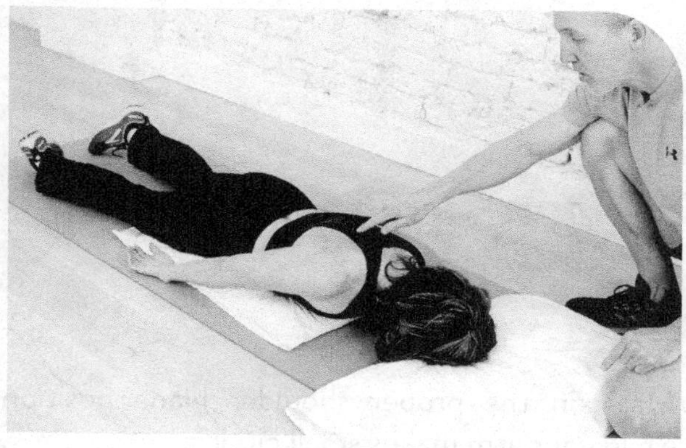

Use a pillow, if needed, to make yourself comfortable.

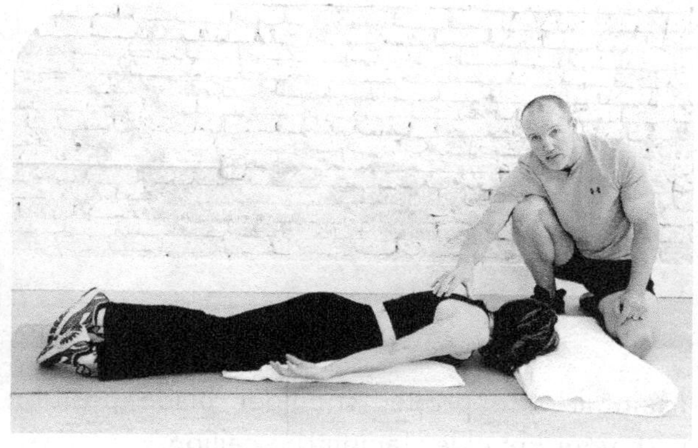

Maintain the proper shoulder blade position.

Videos are available for all exercises and habit changes presented in this book. Go to the website top3fix.com and enter your email and the code TOP3FIX to access them.

• • •

Level 3. Perform Levels 1 and 2. With your hand off the ground, reverse your hand position so that your knuckles face the ceiling, and your palm faces the ground. Maintain the correct shoulder blade position while holding your hand off the ground.

Hold for three breaths, noting how successful or easy this is. Lower your entire arm and shoulder blade together as one unit back to the ground to rest.

Repeat three times. Switch to the other side.

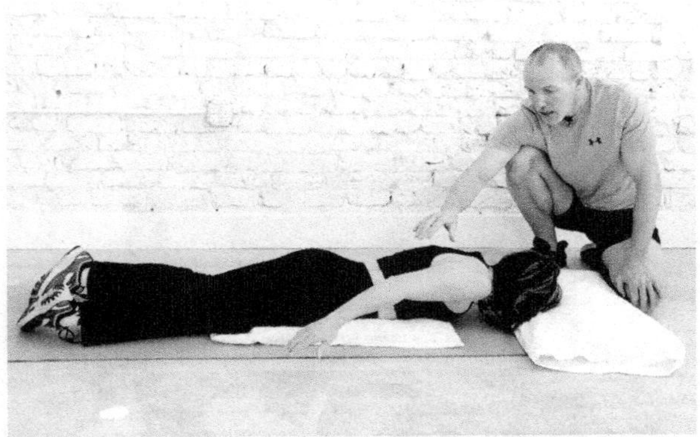

Maintain the proper shoulder blade position with your knuckles facing the ceiling.

Level 4. Perform Levels 1, 2, and 3. With your hand off the ground, move your arm away from your side, eventually achieving an angle of approximately 80 degrees from your body. You may need to begin with an angle of just 10 or 20 degrees from your body. Maintaining this angle, make ten small circles with your arm, with your hand lightly brushing the ground at the bottom of each circle. Reverse the direction of the circles and perform another ten repetitions. Maintain the correct shoulder blade position the entire time your hand is off the ground.

Bring your arm back to your side and lower your entire arm and shoulder blade, together as one unit, back to the ground to rest.

Repeat three times. Switch to the other side.

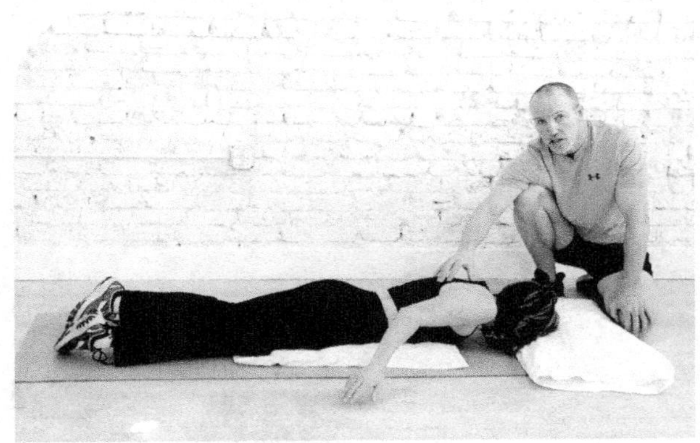

Maintain the proper shoulder blade position while your arm makes small circles.

Chest Stretch

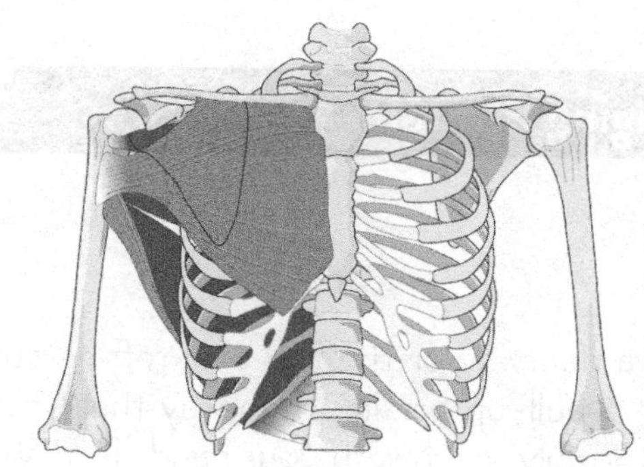

Lie on your back with your knees bent to flatten your lower back against the ground and your arms by your sides with palms facing the ceiling. If you prefer, place a pillow under your head to promote relaxation. Keeping your palms facing up, slide your arms out to the side as if you are making a snow angel until a gentle stretch is felt in your chest, the front of your shoulder and your upper arm. It should not be painful or straining to maintain this position. Hold for 30–60 seconds. Be sure that your lower back does not arch. Return your arms to your sides. Repeat, sliding your arms further if you comfortably can, holding, and returning your arms to your sides. Try to keep your wrists and elbows touching the ground for as long as you can—your elbows will lift from the ground at some point. Notice any asymmetries between your arms.

Eventually, you will be able to bring your arms overhead, with your hands meeting in the middle. Once you achieve this position, try to bring your elbows toward your midline to stretch some of the rotator cuff muscles. Do not allow your lower back to arch off the ground as a way of achieving the arms overhead position.

As this stretch becomes easier, it can be done on a half or full foam roller.

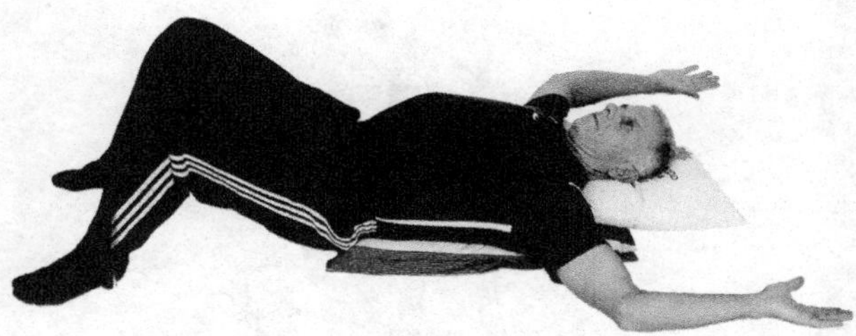

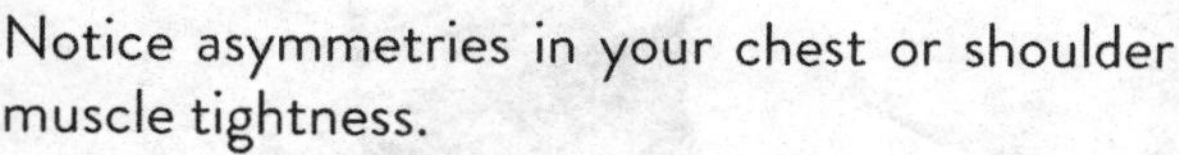

Notice asymmetries in your chest or shoulder muscle tightness.

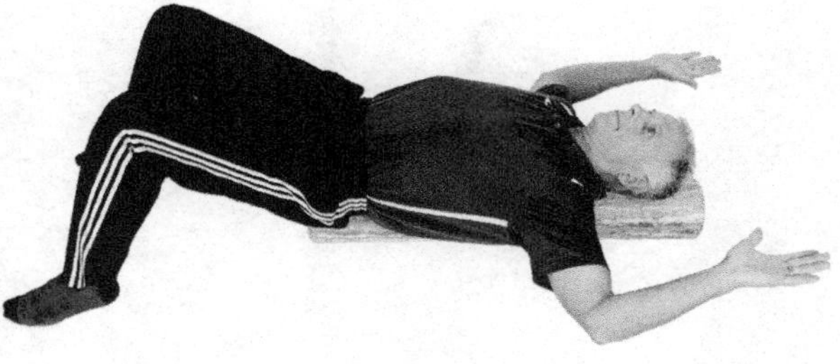

Do not allow your lower back to arch during this stretch.

Hanging Stretch

Find a doorway or the top of a refrigerator or place a pull-up bar in a doorway that you can comfortably reach with your hand. Turn so that you are perpendicular to the door, with your right side closer to the door and your palm facing away from you. Step your right foot into the doorway—this will help support your body weight and reduce strain on your shoulder. Gently lean to the right, feeling the right rib cage stretch. Explore bending your knees a little to accentuate the stretch. Breathe three times into the right rib cage to further assist the muscle lengthening. Return to standing.

Repeat on the left side. Notice any asymmetries in tightness between sides.

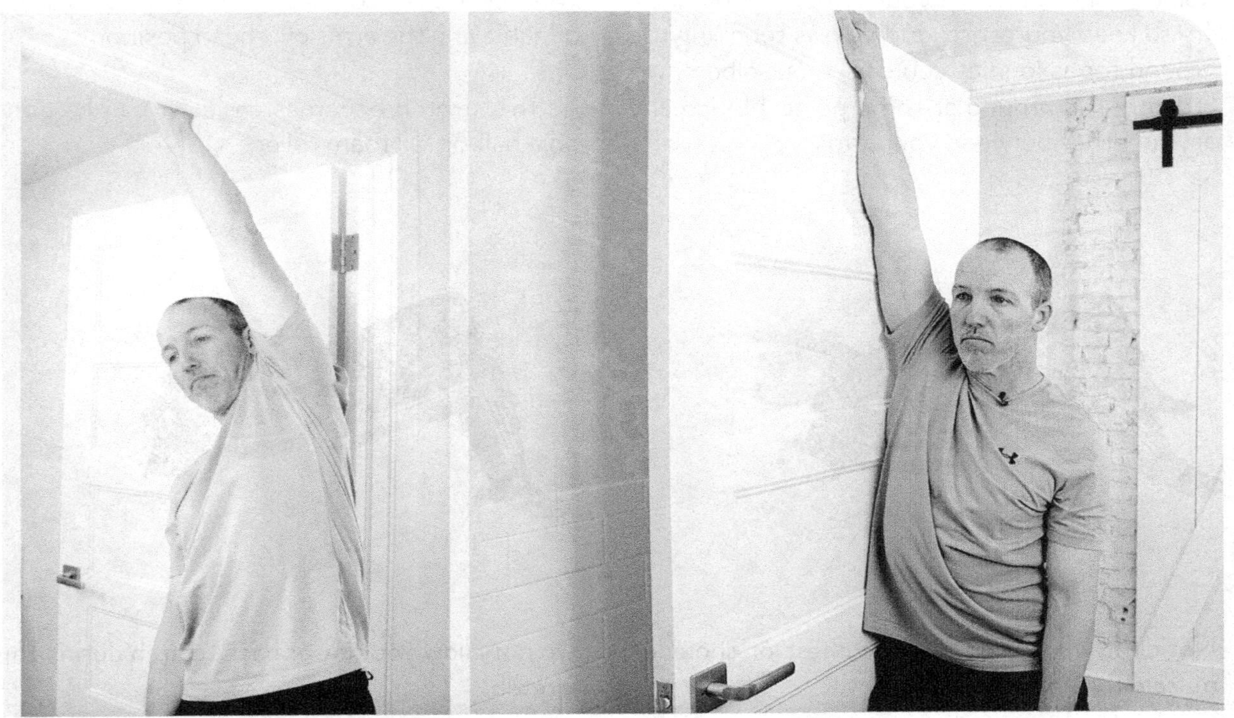

Bear weight through your right leg to reduce stress on your right shoulder.

Fix Pain-Causing Habits

Sleeping

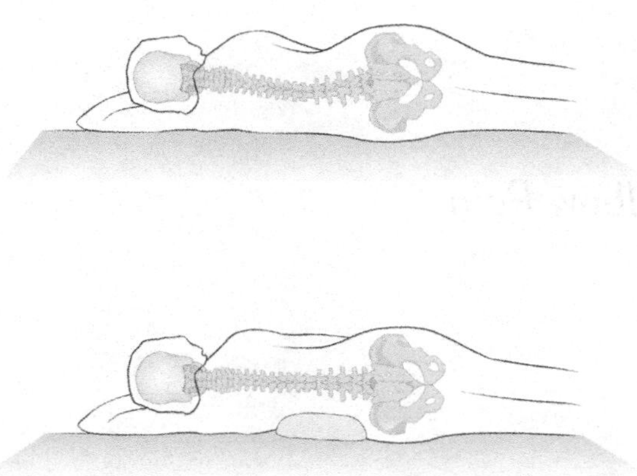

Side sleeping can irritate your shoulders because the shoulders are one of the widest parts of the body, so have more contact pressure with the bed. To reduce this pressure, place a folded towel or pillow under your rib cage. Your rib cage will now bear some of the weight, reducing shoulder pain. You may need to adjust your head pillow height as a result.

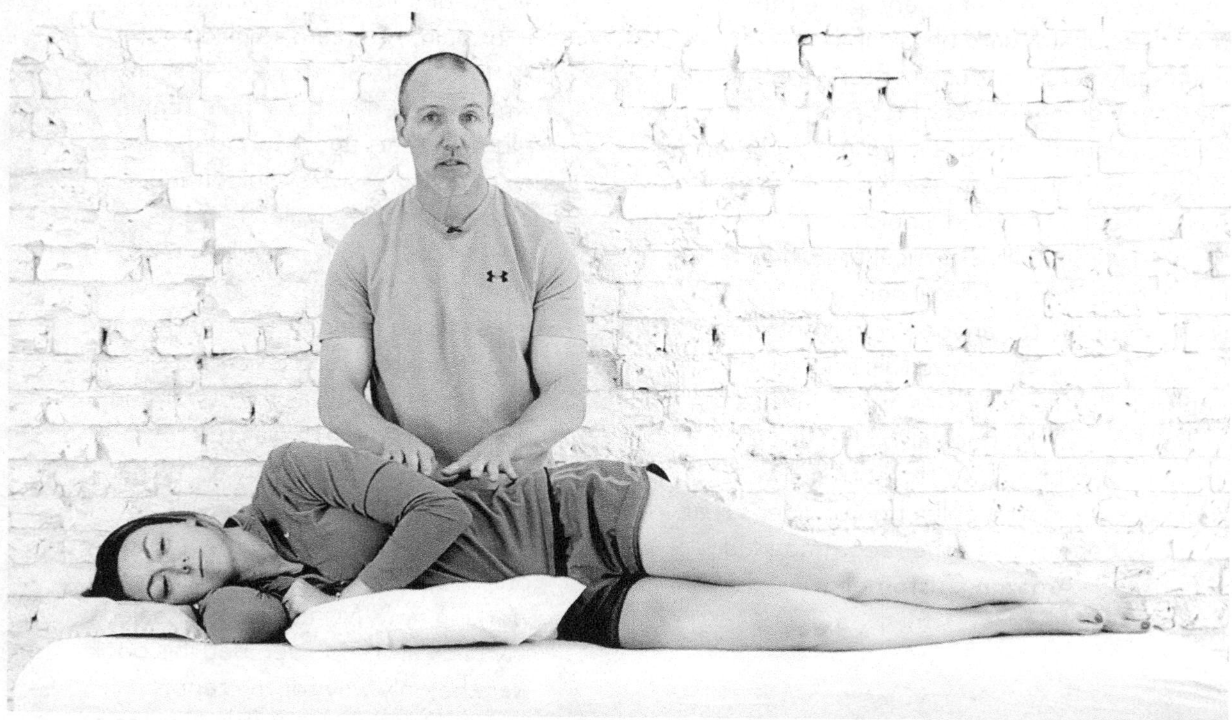

Placing a towel or pillow under your rib cage can help reduce pressure on your shoulder during sleep.

CHAPTER 8

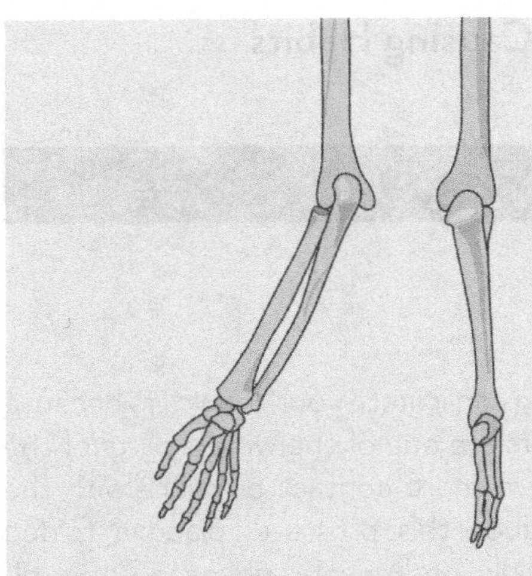

Elbow Pain

"I've spent an awfully large amount of time and money, consumed wheelbarrows full of remedies and ointments, and gone through the paces of standard physical therapy for a previously persistent case of tennis elbow. By simply doing the very first exercise Rick Olderman recommends in *Fixing You: Shoulder & Elbow Pain*, I've experienced relief from pain. After having tried a number of other things, I was initially skeptical that there would be anything new or useful here. All I can do is emphatically tell anyone who is suffering from tennis elbow to give this book, and more importantly, the exercises and stretches within, an honest try. The book also contains a link to an invaluable bonus. At the author's website, there is a wonderful collection of videos that properly demonstrate the recommended exercises." **-Amazon Customer**

"Honestly, you must buy this book if you have had tennis elbow, golfer's elbow or stiff shoulder, epicondylitis, joint pain, RSI. I am so glad I got it. After 5 years of pain and disability which started with a simple tennis elbow 5 years ago, I found the link to my progressive shoulder and elbow pain and swollen hands is ALL CONNECTED! It provides great stretching diagrams and online video links so you can do the stretches and strength exercises. The assisted forearm stretch was my savior and now I am healing. It was the forearm muscles that twisted my arms that were tight, causing golfer's elbow and my right arm to be mechanically out of sync but the exercises are working now. My osteopath healed my back and shoulder, but this book was the only way for my tennis elbow. Recommended!!!! Five stars."
-Amazon Customer

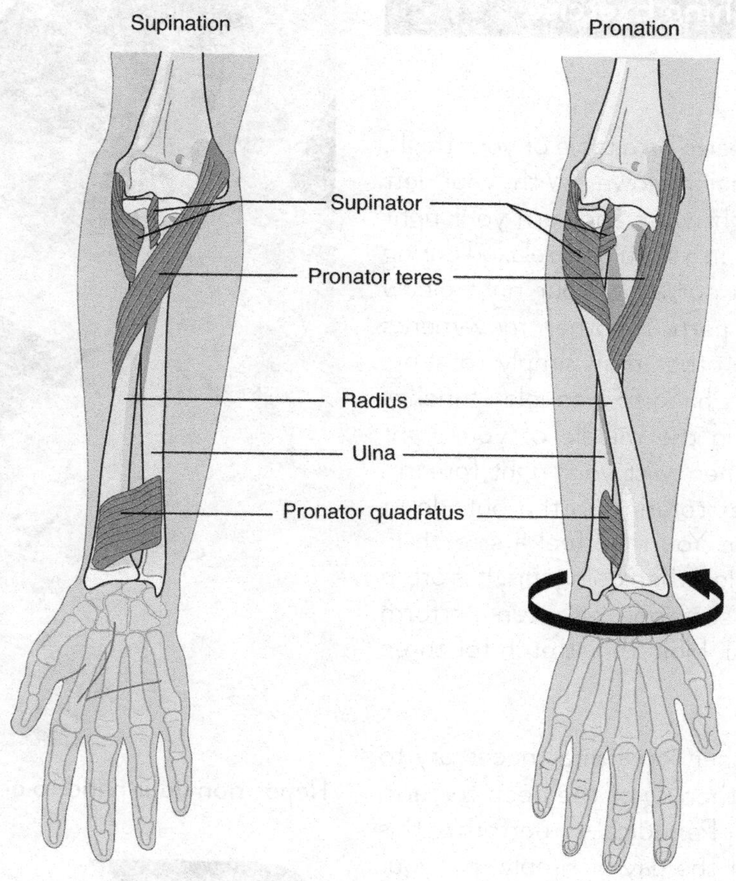

The forearm rotator muscles attach where most tennis or golfer's elbow pain is felt and often become short.

Elbow pain is often caused by tension or shortness of the deeper forearm rotator muscles. These muscles insert precisely where most people experience tennis or golfer's elbow pain. Elbow pain can also be the result of dysfunctional shoulder mechanics. Therefore, consider following the exercises in Chapter 7, Shoulder Pain.

Forearm Stretching Exercise

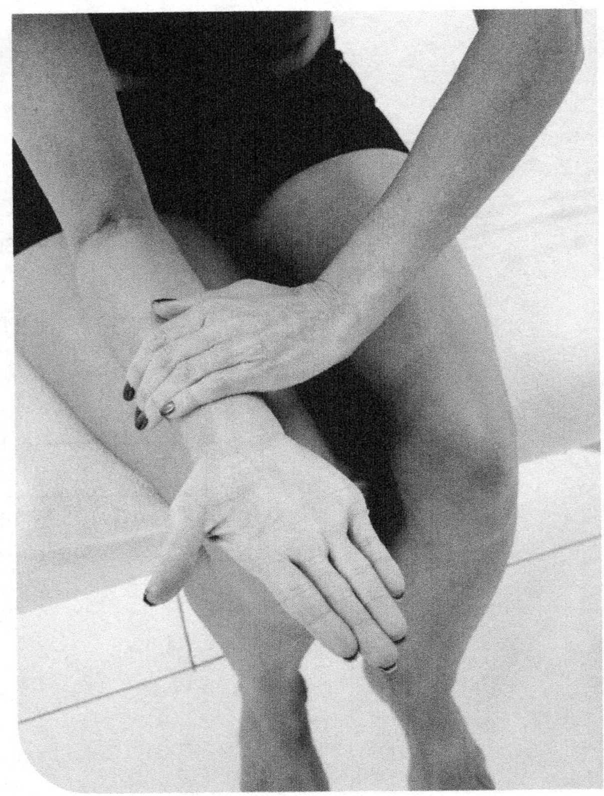

Reposition your hand to create a good stretch.

Rest your right forearm on a table or your thigh, with your palm facing down. With your left hand, hold your right wrist and turn your right palm up. Your right arm should be relaxed during this maneuver. Do not allow your right elbow or upper arm to perform other movements during this stretch other than simply rotating. Reposition your left hand to a couple of inches above your wrist, in the middle of your right forearm. Now further twist your right forearm so that it continues rotating to the outside of your right shoulder. You may feel a stretch in your forearm muscles when doing this. It is often more effective if someone else can perform this stretch for you. Hold the stretch for three breaths.

Repeat on your other forearm as necessary to reinforce this lengthening of the deep forearm rotator muscles. Periodically perform this stretch throughout the day or simply rest your arms in a palms-up position to naturally lengthen these rotator muscles.

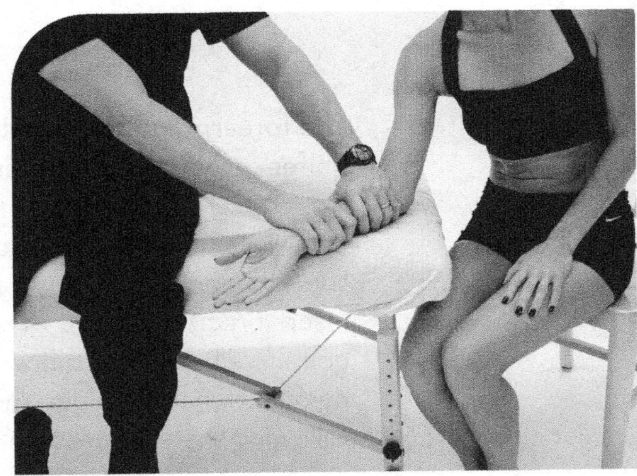

Assistance with this stretch will improve its effectiveness.

• • •

Videos are available for all exercises and habit changes presented in this book. Go to the website top3fix.com and enter your email and the code TOP3FIX to access them.

Self-Brachialis Massage

The brachialis muscle lies beneath the biceps muscle and crosses the elbow joint. This muscle is often irritated with prolonged forearm rotation, as when typing, especially if the arms are not supported correctly. Massaging this muscle has helped many relieve elbow pain.

Simply use your fingers or thumb to locate the cord-like biceps tendon at the elbow. Then, slide your fingers to either side of the tendon to the more sensitive and fleshier brachialis. Gently massage this muscle on both sides of the biceps tendon to relieve strain on the elbow. Tennis elbow sufferers will note more tenderness on the outside of the central biceps tendon, while golfer's elbow sufferers will find more tenderness on the inside of the biceps tendon.

Following the upper body ergonomics recommendations provided in Chapters 4-6 will help to decrease the stress on this muscle and reduce elbow pain.

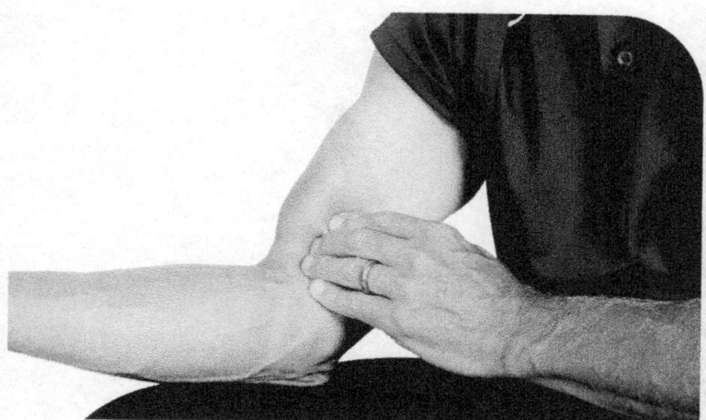

The brachialis muscle becomes strained due to poor ergonomics.

Fix Pain-Causing Habits

Mouse Ergonomics

Many people with chronic elbow pain happen to also use a computer mouse for work. To reduce strain on the elbow, bring the mouse close to your body so that your arm is supported, as mentioned in the upper body ergonomics recommendations in Chapters 4-6. If you use a mouse often, move your keyboard to the side to make the location of the mouse more central in your workstation.

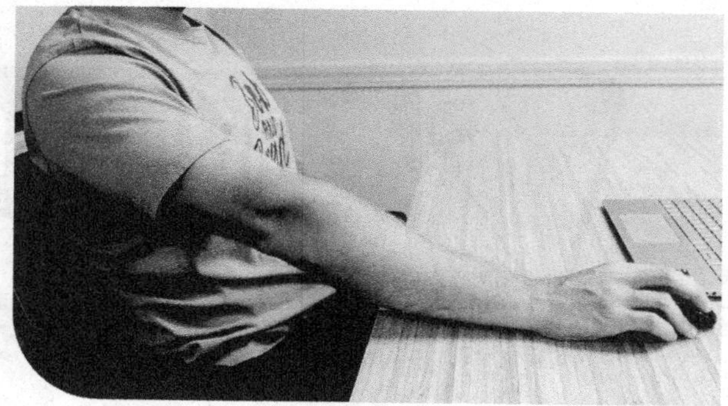

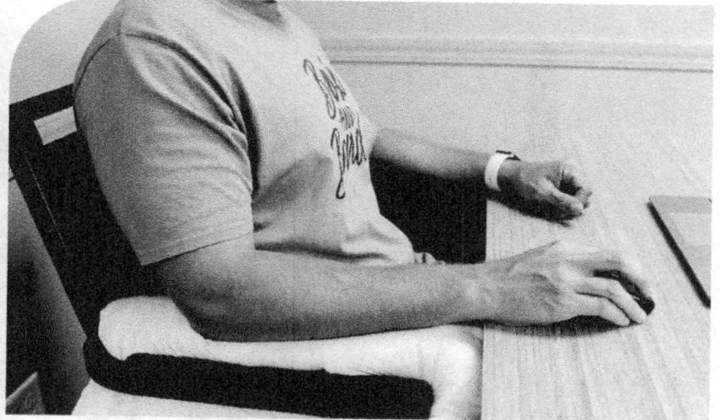

Bring your mouse closer to you to reduce elbow strain.

SECTION 2

THE LOWER BODY SYSTEM

CHAPTER 9

How the Lower Body System Works

This chapter will lay the foundation for understanding what the lower body system is and how it works in relation to the pelvis and spine. We will continue to keep the discussion simple, providing the broad strokes of how it all fits together. To learn in more detail about the muscles, bones, and biomechanics of this system, please read my books *Fixing You: Back Pain, 2nd Edition*, *Fixing You: Hip & Knee Pain*, *Fixing You: Foot & Ankle Pain*, and *Fixing You: Back Pain During Pregnancy*.

The information in this section will help you solve the following conditions:

- -Two-Sided (Central) Back Pain
- -One-Sided Back Pain
- -Sciatica
- -Spondylolisthesis
- -Stenosis
- -Sacroiliac Joint Pain
- -Piriformis Pain
- -Hip Pain
- -Knee Pain
- -Plantar Fasciitis

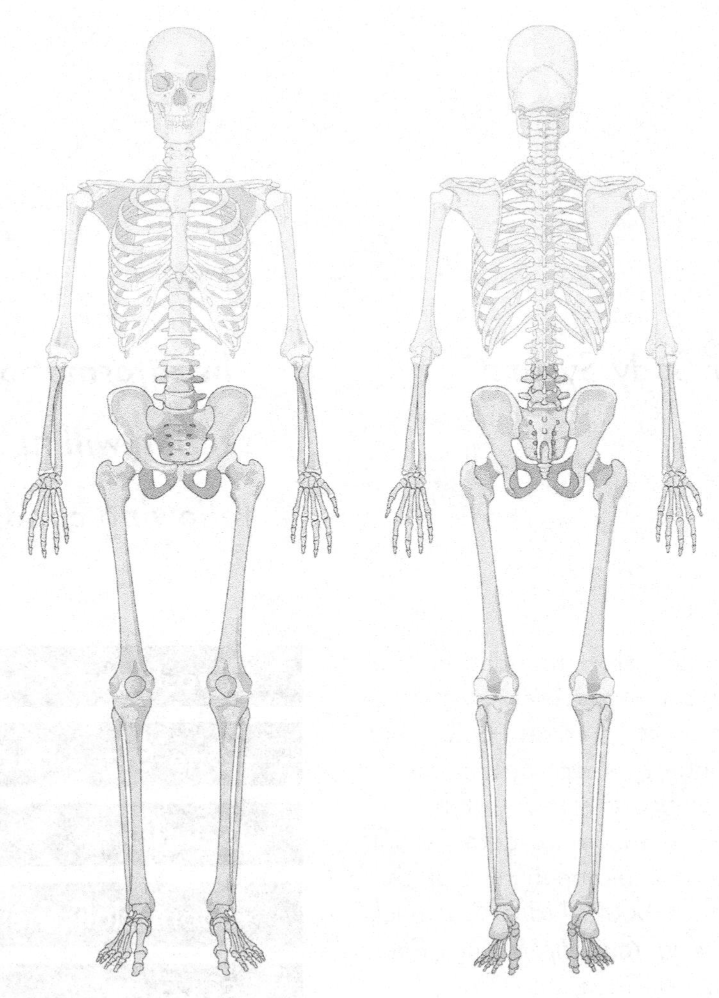

The pelvis is the center of function of the lower body system.

Just as the shoulder blade is the center of function for the upper body system, the pelvis is the center of function for the lower body and back system.

Cervical vertebrae (C1-C7)
Thoracic vertebrae (T1-T12)
Lumbar vertebrae (L1-L5)
Kyphotic curve
Lordotic curve

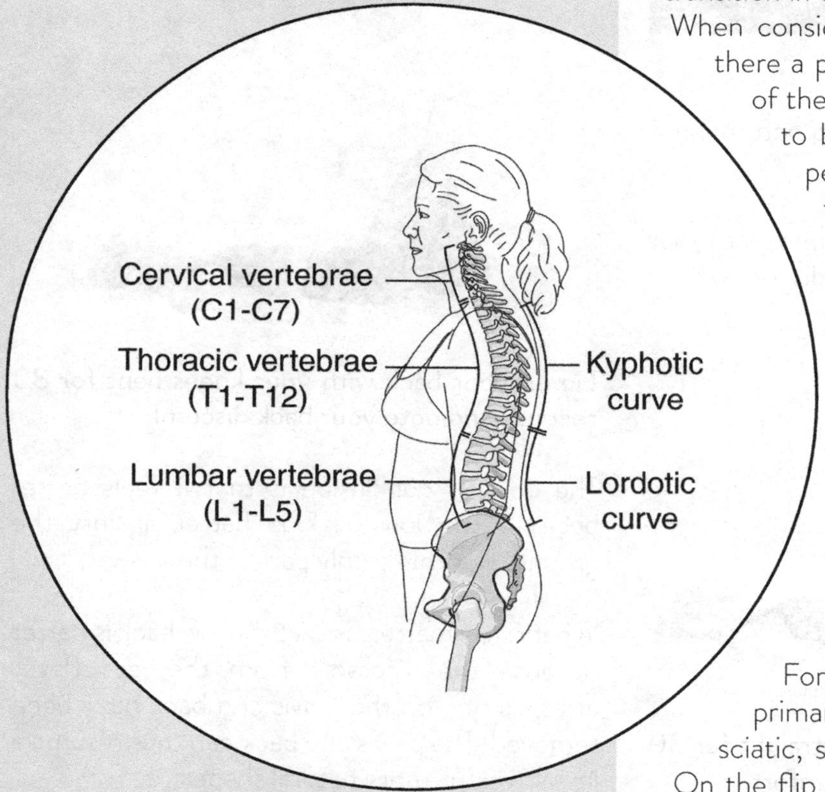

Transitions in the curves of the spine are natural stress points.

If you look closely at the spine, you will notice several curves. The points at which these curves transition in direction are natural stress points. When considering the low back, not only is there a pronounced curve at the junction of the pelvis and lower spine, causing it to be susceptible to stress, but the pelvis is also highly mobile, adding further potential strain to this vulnerability.

Now consider that the legs are quite long and are very active when performing activities such as walking, running, or exercising. The legs (and the muscles attaching the legs to the pelvis) are significant lever arms acting on the pelvis and therefore on the spine.

For this reason, the legs are the primary culprits behind chronic back, sciatic, sacroiliac joint, or piriformis pain. On the flip side, they are also the heroes in solving these types of pain.

Two broad patterns of problems cause most chronic back and pelvic pain: **Extension Problems** and **Sidebending Problems.**

Extension Problems

An Extension Problem is present if pain is exacerbated when the spine is arched or extended.

Extension Problem Test

Here's an easy test to perform to determine if you have an Extension Problem.

Step 1. Lie on your back for 30 seconds with your legs straight. Note your low back discomfort.

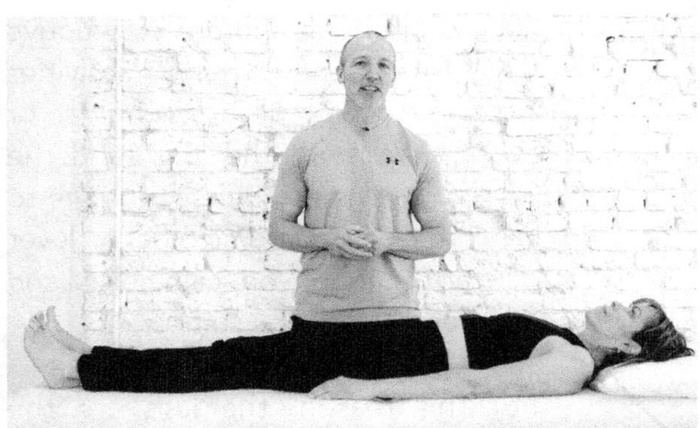

Lie on your back with your legs straight for 30 seconds and note your back discomfort.

Step 2. Bend your knees so that your feet are flat on the ground or hug your knees to your chest.

Which of the two positions (legs straight or knees bent) feel better for your back? Nearly 100% of those reading this book will find that their back feels better when their knees are bent.

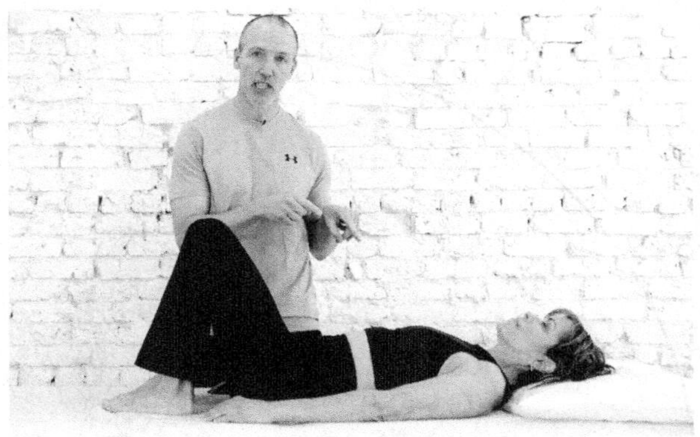

Lie on your back with your knees bent for 30 seconds and note your back discomfort.

The obvious conclusion is that it feels better because the low back is flatter against the ground. But this is only part of the answer.

What really matters is that the low back is flatter because the stressors from the legs (lever arms) acting on the pelvis and back have been removed. The pelvis and back can thus resume a less stressful, more natural shape.

What's amazing is relief can often be felt instantly, regardless of whether herniated discs, bulging discs, arthritic changes, stenosis, spondylolisthesis, disc degeneration, nerve root compression, or any other type of structural problem that showed up on an X-ray or MRI are present. Essentially, you've just experienced how good your back could feel if you simply removed the stressors from your legs that are acting on it!

Sidebending Problems

The second pattern of problems, which leads to most cases of one-sided back pain, sciatica, sacroiliac joint pain, or piriformis syndrome, is a Sidebending Problem.

A Sidebending Problem occurs when one side of the pelvis is higher than the other side. Typically, the rib cage on the same side is lower. Naturally, this creates more compression on that side of the spine and compromises the sciatic nerve roots.

This pattern is often mistaken for a leg-length discrepancy, but a true leg-length discrepancy is likely not the issue. Instead, it's a functional compensation pattern due to an older lower body problem on the same side of the elevated pelvis in 80%–90% of cases, or a compensation pattern from the opposite leg in 10%–20% of cases.

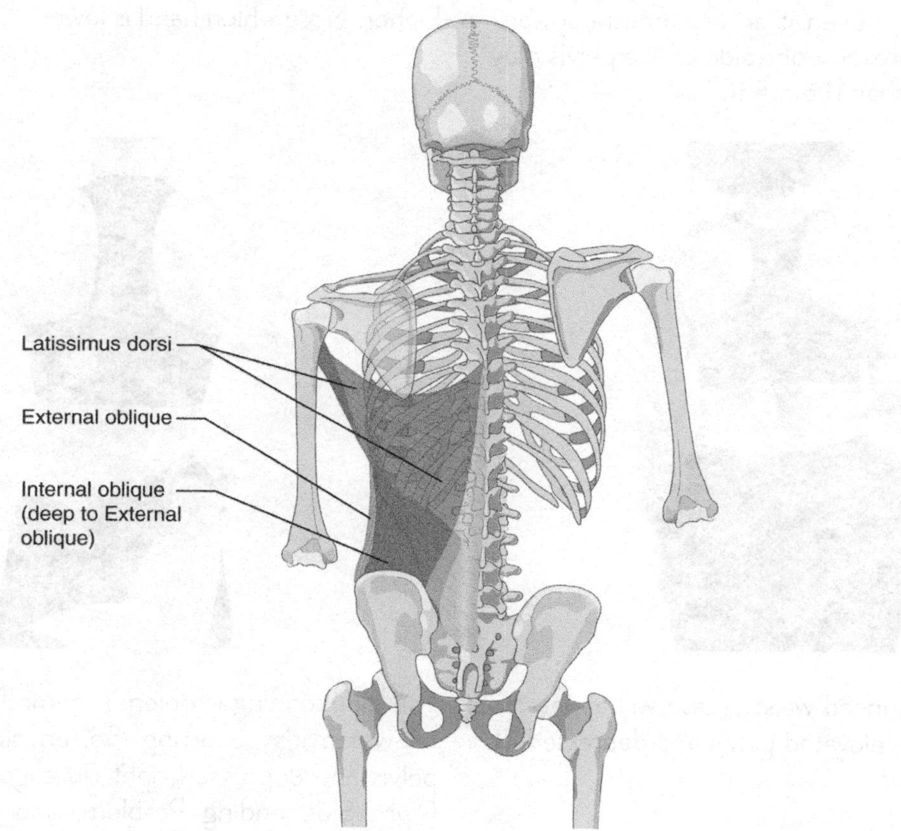

A Sidebending Problem typically consists of an elevated pelvis on one side together with a depressed rib cage on the same side.

Sidebending Problem Test

A simple way to determine if you have a Sidebending Problem is to remove your shirt and take a picture of your back. A larger waist crease on one side is typically present when there is a Sidebending Problem. This is the side with the elevated pelvis and depressed rib cage—the side of compression. That crease will likely correspond to the side of pain or to some older leg injury. Even if an asymmetrical waist crease is not present, one side of the pelvis may still be higher than the other.

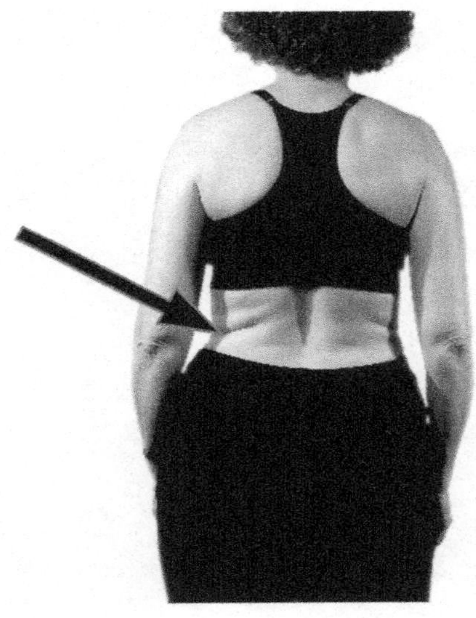

A more pronounced waist crease will appear on the side of the elevated pelvis and depressed rib cage.

A more precise way to test for a Sidebending Problem is to measure the height of the iliac crests of the pelvis. The tester places their hands on the very top of the iliac crests, making sure to avoid the outsides of the iliac crests, by pushing into the fleshy part of the waist and feeling the bony iliac crests under their hands. Note which hand is higher.

From here, feel just above the iliac crests, toward the head, and find the bottom of the rib cage. It will be very close to the iliac crests and will likely be lower on the same side on which the pelvis is higher. Note which hand is lower.

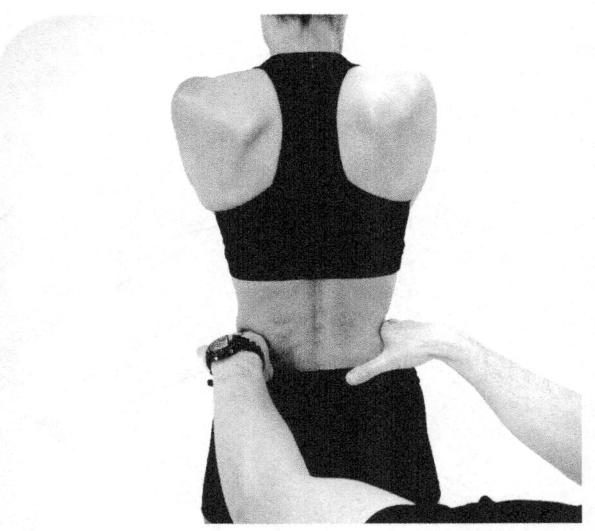

The Sidebending Problem is named for the side on which it's occurring. So, an elevated right pelvis and depressed right rib cage would be a Right Sidebending Problem, and an elevated left pelvis and depressed left rib cage would be a Left Sidebending Problem.

Solve Your Sidebending Problem Rapidly

An elevated right pelvis and depressed left rib cage indicate a Complex Sidebending Problem. This is a hallmark of congenital scoliosis, which often causes an S-shaped curvature of the spine. It can be thought of as a spine with two Sidebending Problems stacked on top of each other.

Fortunately, Sidebending Problems can be solved easily.

In medicine, the term "scoliosis" simply indicates a lateral curve in the spine. Based on this definition, most people have scoliosis. But it's important to realize that a Sidebending Problem is a functional form of scoliosis that creates a single curve in the spine and is typically correctible. Congenital scoliosis, two lateral curves creating an S-curve, is rarer and shouldn't be confused with functional scoliosis. These curves can also be treated but create unique issues in the trunk.

To quickly level the pelvis and rib cage if you are someone with a Right Sidebending Problem, raise your right hand in the air and walk for 10–20 steps. Bring your arm back down and remeasure the pelvis and rib cage. They will likely be perfectly level.

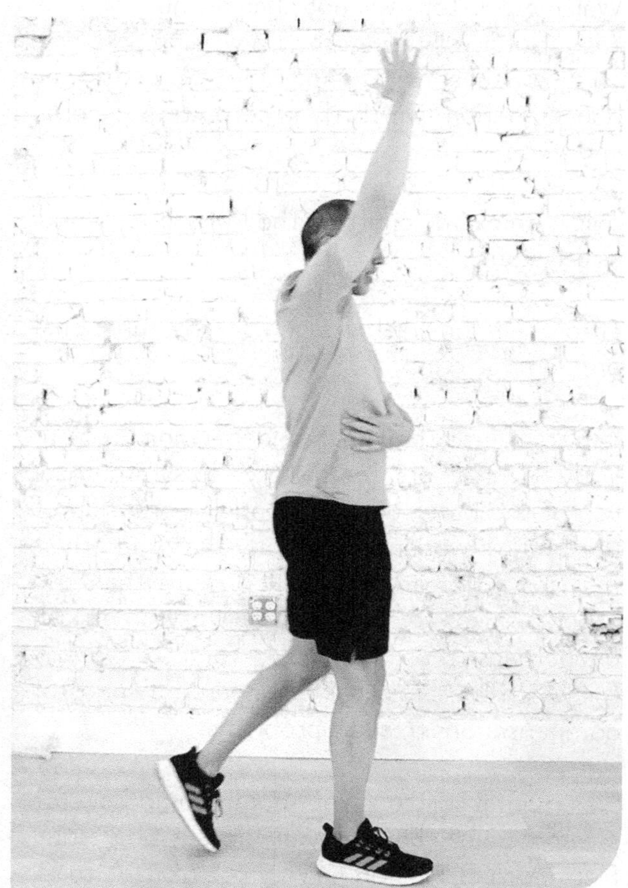

Walk with your arm raised to temporarily correct a Sidebending Problem.

Note: The waist crease will not instantly disappear because the skin, fat, and fascial tissues have adapted to the Sidebending Problem.

For many people, this can seem like a miracle! But once you understand how the body works as a system, you'll come to expect these types of rapid changes in function and pain.

This correction is proof of the absence of a leg-length discrepancy at the root of this pattern. Walking 20 steps will not change the length of a leg. But it will help correct a walking problem. This maneuver will temporarily improve lower body function, which then corrects the pelvis and spine.

This is an example of how the lower body works as a system.

Throw out the heel lifts and fix the functional problems instead!

It makes sense, then, that a Sidebending Problem likely has its roots in a history of asymmetrical use of the lower body. Essentially, one side of the body is working differently than the other. Perhaps you lean on one leg more than the other, perhaps your workstation is asymmetrical, or perhaps there's an old, forgotten injury for which the brain has engineered a series of compensations to avoid problems.

This mental jiujitsu is very common and occurs subconsciously because our focus is on getting from A to B, not on *how* to get from A to B. Therefore, when using the exercises in this section, pay special attention to asymmetries between the two legs. Often, solving the discrepancies solves the pain.

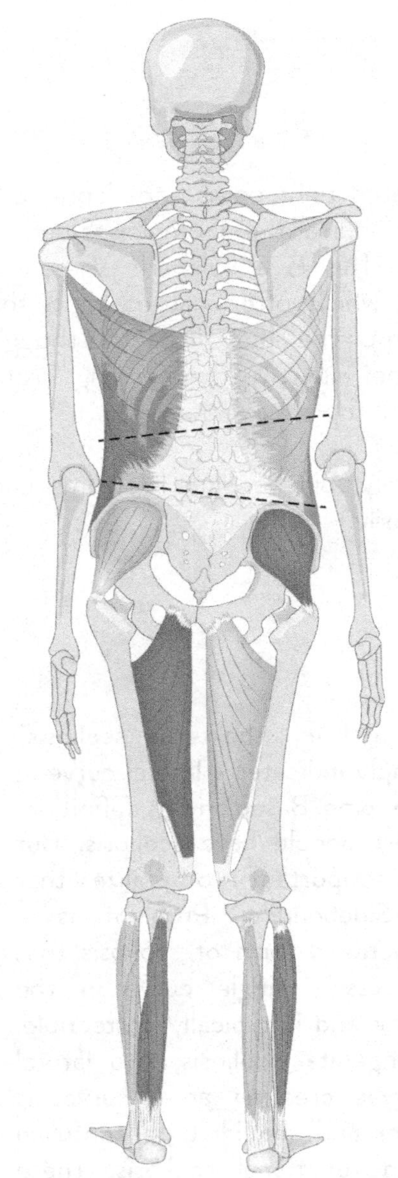

The brain makes subtle subconscious adjustments to work around mechanical obstacles.

People can have both an Extension and Sidebending Problem occur at the same time. In the case of one-sided back, sciatic, sacroiliac joint, or piriformis pain, this is very likely.

Walking

While walking is a good form of exercise, walking poorly is not, and it actually causes pain. If you were able to correct your Sidebending Problem using the walking method with your hand in the air (above), you now have an appreciation for the profound effects that walking mechanics have on the pelvis and spine.

When walking, most people make two very large errors: their knees lock straight and their body lags behind the advancing foot when the foot strikes the ground.

When both problems occur, key lower body muscles are turned off and, consequently, others are excessively turned on. If you're interested in learning more, please refer to my book, *Fixing You: Back Pain*, 2nd Edition.

CLIENT CONNECTION

Recently, I helped a woman who'd had to leave her collegiate swimming program 15 years earlier due to back pain that none of her Division 1 school medical professionals, nor anyone since, had been able to solve. She actually came in for severe plantar fasciitis in both feet that had been unrelenting for months. She'd given up on finding anyone who could solve her back pain. She was in so much pain that she needed about 30 seconds to recover when changing body positions from sitting to standing or lying down. I couldn't even conduct an exam. Fortunately, because I understand the body as a system and how important gait is for lower body system health, I saw the problem just by watching her walk to my table. I instructed her to unlock her knees while walking or standing until I saw her again—that was it. Three days later, a different person entered my clinic. She was smiling and walking without significant pain—her back and plantar fasciitis were 75% better!

This highlights why walking correctly will be a central behavior common to all solutions presented in this book for the lower body system.

Let's get started solving your pain.

CHAPTER 10

Two-Sided (Central) Low Back Pain

"Buy this book, do what it says, and you will be thankful the rest of your life for Rick Olderman. If your back hurts—it's the only book you need." **-Amazon Customer**

"I've had back pain since 2005. I've had two nerve blocks, four injections, numerous doctor visits, pain management clinics, and not one of them has ever helped me with pain or took the time to explain anything structurally to me, until I ran across this book! Learning about your body and changing a few simple things will shift your body and rid your pain. This book is life-changing no matter what the cause of your back issue is." **-Amazon Customer**

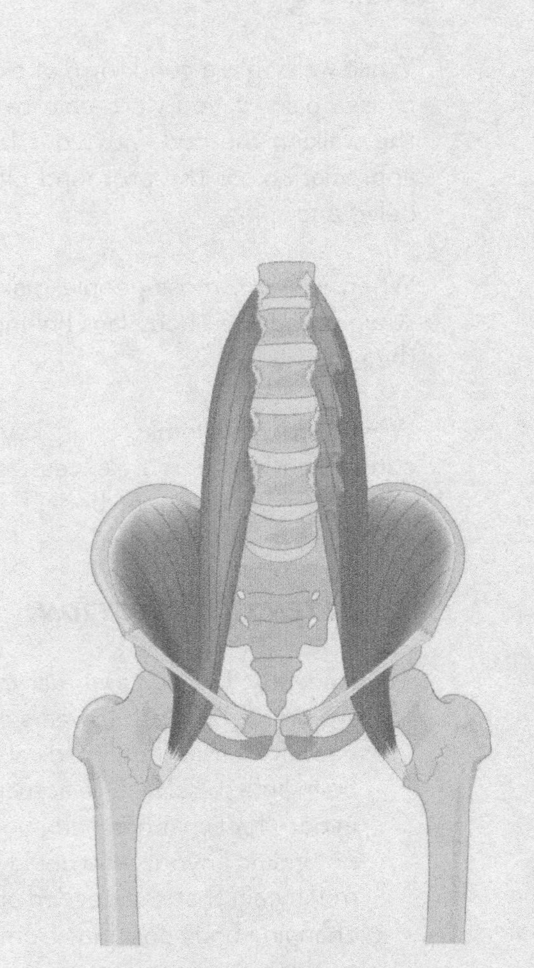

The focus of these exercises is to reduce the forces pulling the spine into more of an arched, or extended, position. Pay special attention to asymmetries in strength, control, and range of motion. Your goals should include moving toward symmetry between the two legs.

Thigh Stretch

On a stable surface, such as a firm table or countertop, lie on your back with both knees drawn to your chest. Place a pillow under your head for additional comfort. Hold both knees with both hands to set your back and relax your legs.

Now, adjust your hands so they are both holding only your left knee. Slowly lower your right foot off the edge of the surface, keeping your right knee bent 90 degrees. Pull your left knee even closer to your chest to prevent your pelvis from rolling forward and your back from arching as you lower your right leg down.

You should feel a stretch in your right upper thigh. Feel your leg gradually lower further as your muscles lengthen, but do not force your right leg down. If you have knee pain, move your right leg out so that your right knee is outside of your right hip. Over time, as your muscles lengthen, gradually move your leg back to the midline. Ideally, your right thigh should be able to rest on the surface with your knee bent 90 degrees and positioned in line with your hip and shoulder. Hold for 7–10 breaths.

Bring your right leg back up to your chest and hug both knees to reset your back and pelvis. Repeat on the left side. Perform twice per side. Repeat 2–3 times per day.

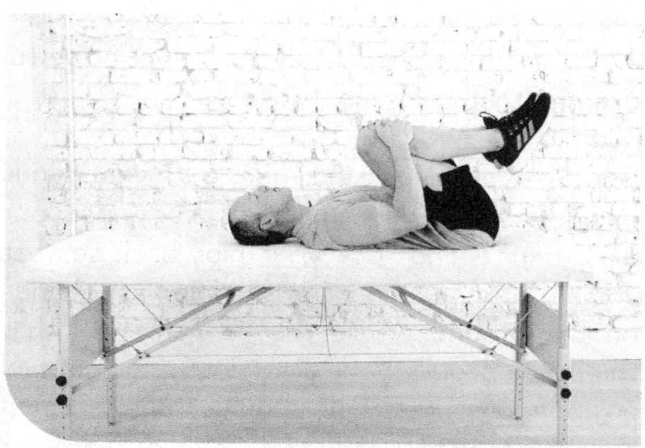

Hug both knees to your chest to set your back and pelvis.

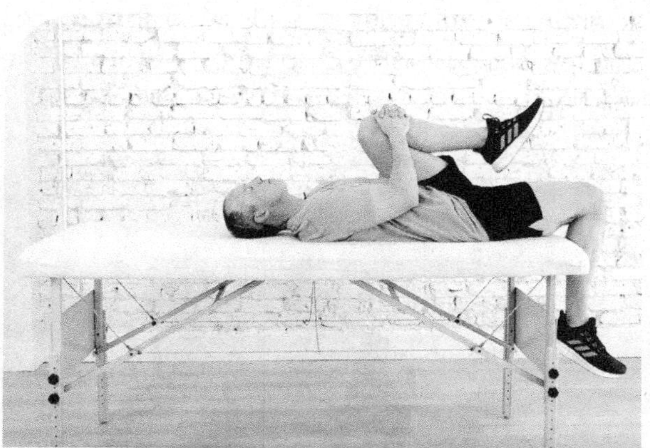

Hold your opposite knee close to your chest to protect your back and pelvis.

All-Fours Rocking Stretch

This exercise passively restores normal hip and low back mechanics while lengthening key muscles that cause back, sciatic, or sacroiliac joint pain. It is a deceptively simple yet powerful exercise that yields big results.

Begin on your hands and knees, with your hands under your shoulders and your knees under your hips. Exhale and rock your hips back so that you are sitting on your feet, keeping your hands on the ground where they began. Feel that this motion pulls your arms into an overhead position. Visualize your shoulder blades being pulled up toward the top of your head. Slide your hands forward, if you are able, to accentuate this stretch. Feel free to rest your head on a small pillow, if you prefer, for support. Feel a nice stretch through your shoulders or armpit area and low back. Breathe 3–5 times. Return to the starting position. Perform 3–5 repetitions.

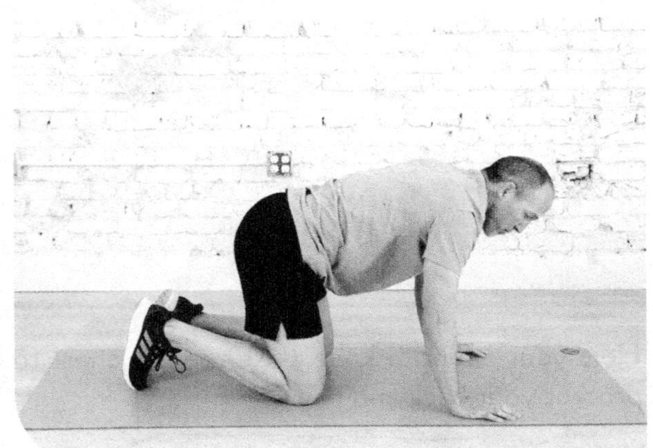

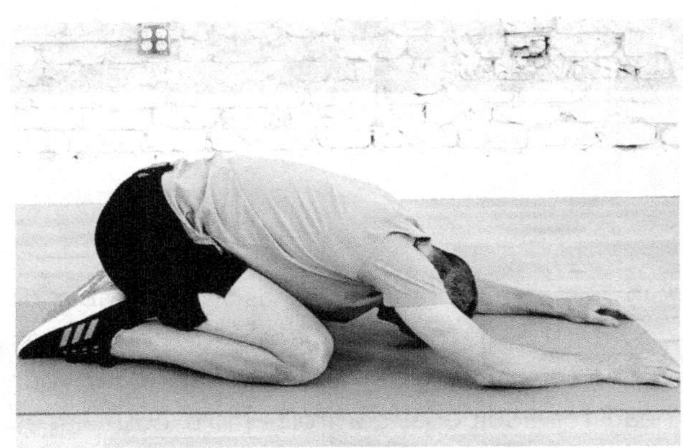

You should feel a stretch in your shoulders, chest, or arms during this exercise.

Take this stretch up a notch after sitting back on your heels by walking both hands to the left. Take three breaths and then walk your hands to the right. If your neck, shoulder, or headache pain is on one side, for example the right side, you'll likely find that your right shoulder and rib cage feel tighter. Solving that tightness will help solve your pain.

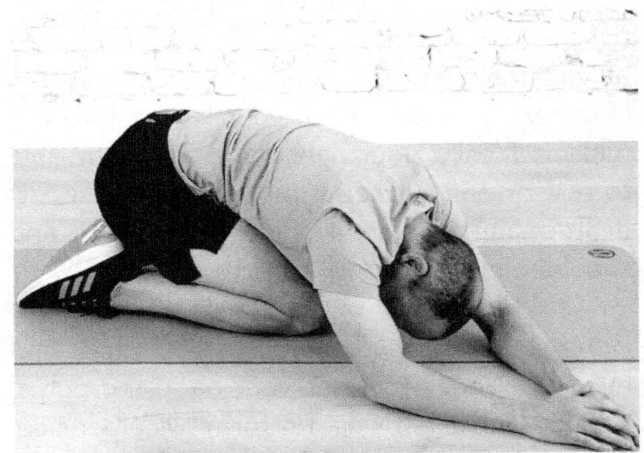

Sidebending while stretching can help you solve unilateral tightness contributing to your pain.

Butt Pumps

Assume a position on your elbows and knees with your lower spine flat, not sagging down toward the ground. Hold your lower spine in place by drawing in your belly button. Use your gluteals (butt muscles) to raise one leg in the air, with your knee bent 90 degrees. Stop at the point at which you feel the maximal contraction of your butt muscles. Do not overuse your low back or hamstring muscles to lift your leg.

Perform a small pump of your leg up and down (about 1–2 inches) while maintaining the gluteal contraction. Do not lower your leg so far that you feel your gluteal muscles turn off; they should remain activated throughout the exercise. Perform 10–30 repetitions, until your gluteals fatigue. Be sure not to recruit your back or hamstring muscles when performing this exercise.

If you don't feel your butt muscles contracting, rotate your knee out slightly until you do, and then perform the pump. Switch sides. Perform two sets per session. Perform 2–3 times per day.

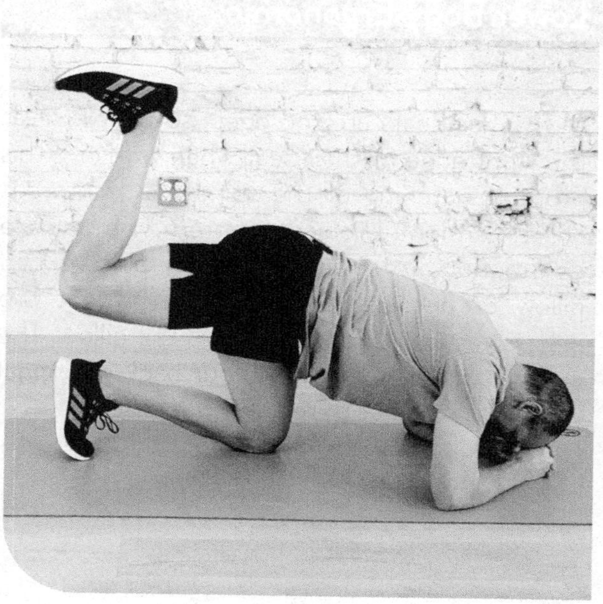

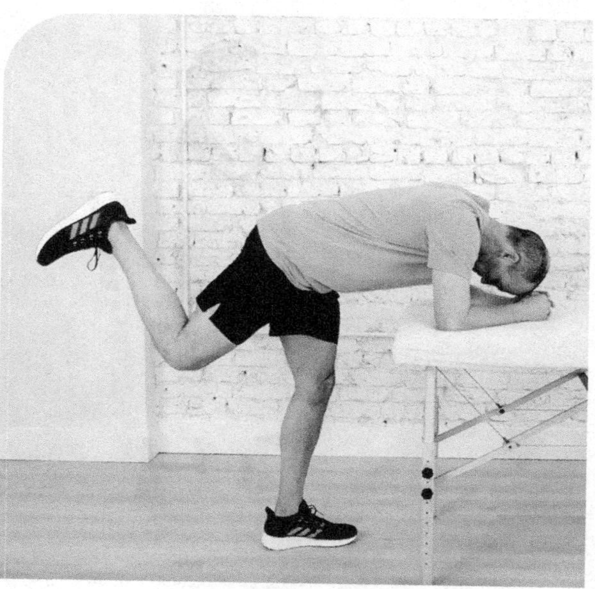

Gluteal strengthening is often the key to most lower body or back pain problems.

• • •

Videos are available for all exercises and habit changes presented in this book. Go to the website top3fix.com and enter your email and the code TOP3FIX to access them.

Fix Pain-Causing Habits

Lower Body Ergonomics

Most chair seats are too deep, so people sit at the front edge of their seat when working. This promotes arching of the spine and reinforces an Extension Problem pattern of muscle contraction. To solve this, simply place a bed pillow or two behind your back. Orient the pillows vertically. Lean back into the pillow. The contact of the pillow with your back will signal your back muscles to relax.

Additionally, place a box under your feet, to raise your knees higher than your hip joints. This will gently roll your pelvis back, flattening your spine.

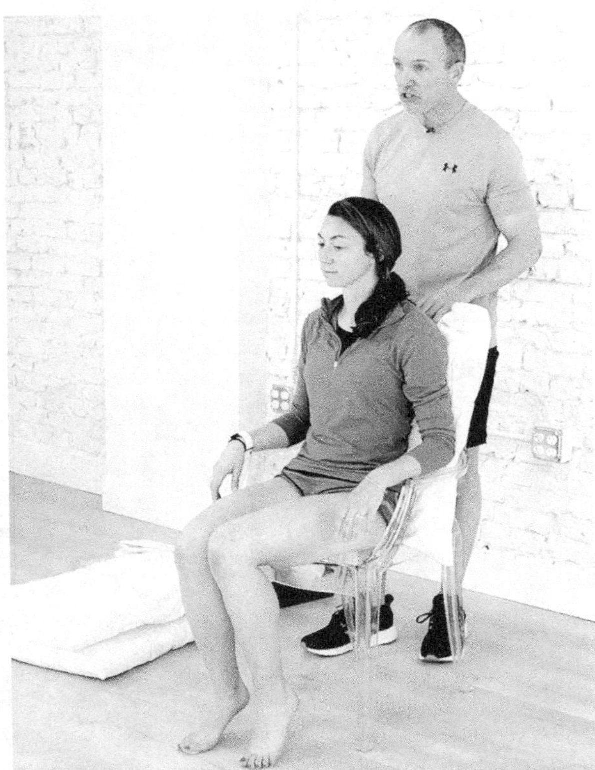

Placing pillows in the back of your chair will signal your back muscles to relax.

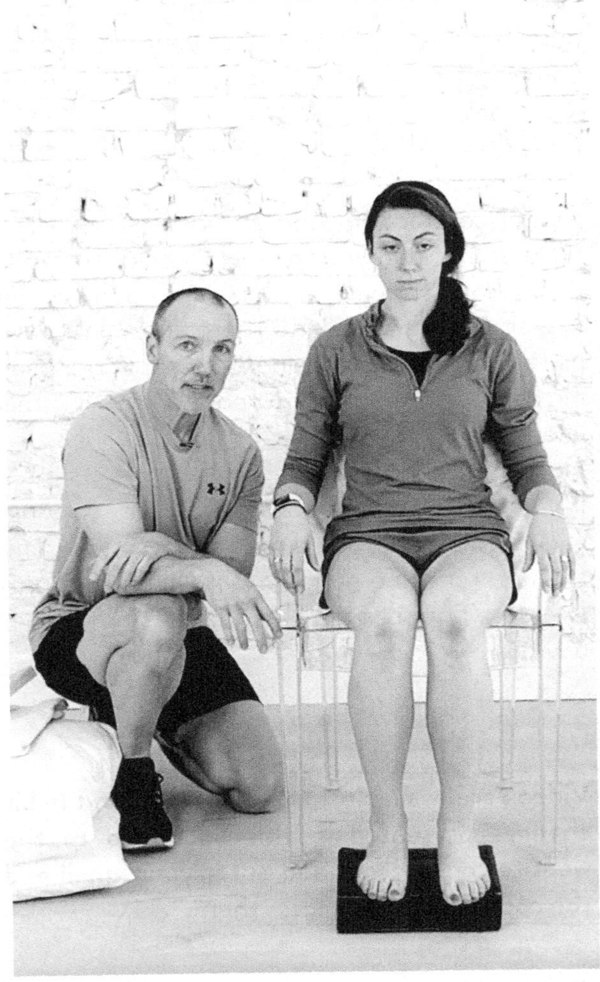

Adding support under your feet helps to tilt your pelvis back and flatten your spine.

Gluteal Walking: Ice-Skating

Pretend you are ice-skating by taking a small lunge forward and slightly out to the side (like a hockey player) with your right leg, bending your knee and leaning forward slightly. Your weight should be mostly on your forward right leg. Pump twice up and down with your forward leg.

Place your hand on your right butt muscle and feel that it becomes firmer with this action. If your butt muscle does not become firmer, bend deeper at your knee and trunk until it does. Now step your left foot forward and repeat with your left leg. Continue for 10–20 steps, gradually straightening your trunk and forward leg until you reach an upright position, with your knee almost straight. You will likely notice that your butt muscles turn off at some point, as you straighten up. Continue practicing until, with your trunk in a fully upright position, you feel natural gluteal activation when your forward foot strikes the ground.

Once you are in a tall, upright position, gradually return to a "normal"-looking walk but with your gluteal muscles activating naturally (not consciously) with each foot strike.

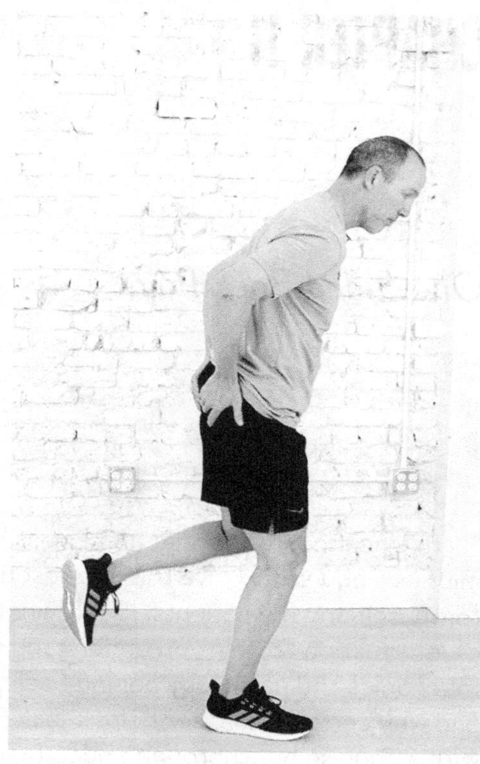

Mimicking ice-skating is a good way to activate your gluteal muscles to prepare for walking.

Gluteal Walking: Tiptoe Walking

Walk on your tiptoes for about 20 steps with your hands on your butt muscles. Feel that your butt muscles contract at each foot strike. This is not a conscious contraction but is instead one that occurs naturally. Then, slowly lower your heels back down and feel that your butt muscles continue to contract naturally as you take steps. Repeat throughout the day until, without needing to tiptoe walk first, you can walk with your gluteal muscles turning on naturally at each foot strike.

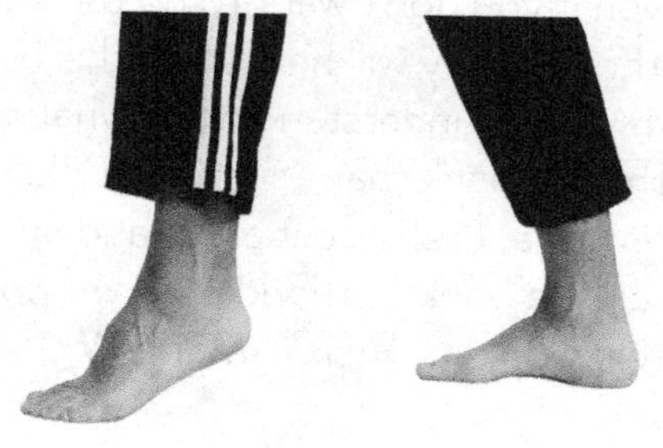

Tiptoe walking is a good way to activate your gluteal muscles to prepare for walking.

CHAPTER 11

One-Sided Back Pain

“I am a healthcare provider and I treat back injuries frequently. I love this as a resource for myself and my patients. It contains a lot of information to help you understand the mechanics and pathology behind back pain and why certain exercises help. It leaves you with a concise but thorough understanding of why you have pain and what to do about it. It is empowering and it works! Rick is a masterful physical therapist and I have every confidence in his advice!” **-Amazon Customer**

“Even if you don’t want to do the exercises (although they will help you), this book will give you an understanding of what’s going on with your back that you may not have seen elsewhere. I refer to it again and again. I’ve given the book to friends and will continue to refer people to Rick.” **-Marie W**

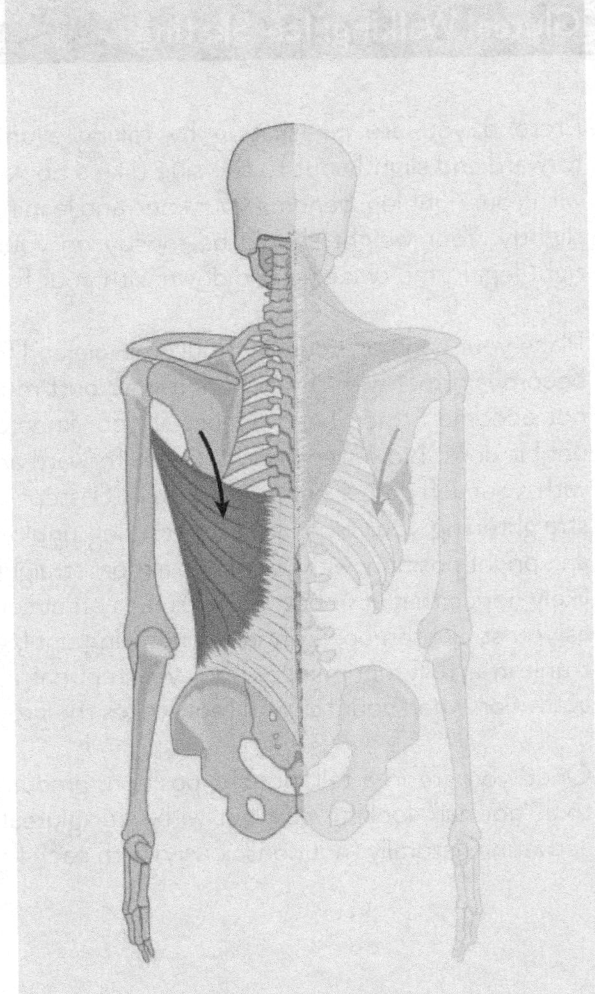

Pay special attention to asymmetries in strength, control, and range of motion during these exercises. Your goals should include moving toward symmetry between the two legs.

Thigh Stretch

On a stable surface, such as a firm table or countertop, lie on your back with both knees drawn to your chest. Place a pillow under your head for additional comfort. Hold both knees with both hands to set your back and relax your legs.

Now, adjust your hands so they are both holding only your left knee. Slowly lower your right foot off the edge of the surface, keeping your right knee bent 90 degrees. Pull your left knee even closer to your chest to prevent your pelvis from rolling forward and your back from arching as you lower your right leg down.

You should feel a stretch in your right upper thigh. Feel your leg gradually lower further as your muscles lengthen, but do not force your right leg down. If you have knee pain, move your right leg out so that your right knee is outside of your right hip. Over time, as your muscles lengthen, gradually move your leg back to the midline. Ideally, your right thigh should be able to rest on the surface, with your knee bent 90 degrees and positioned in line with your hip and shoulder. Hold for 7–10 breaths.

Bring your right leg back up to your chest and hug both knees to reset your back and pelvis. Repeat on the left side. Perform twice per side. Repeat 2–3 times per day.

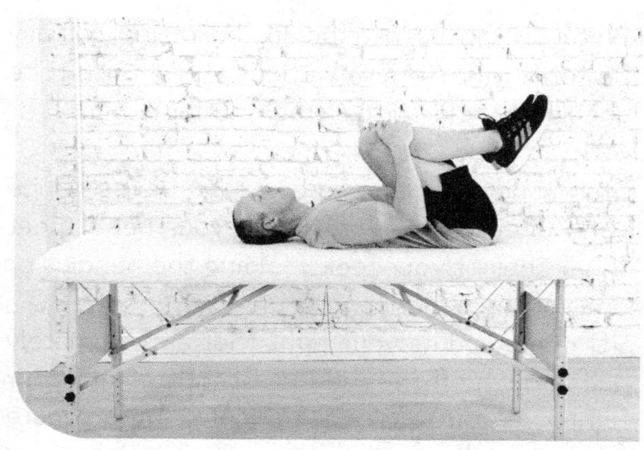

Hug both knees to your chest to set your back and pelvis.

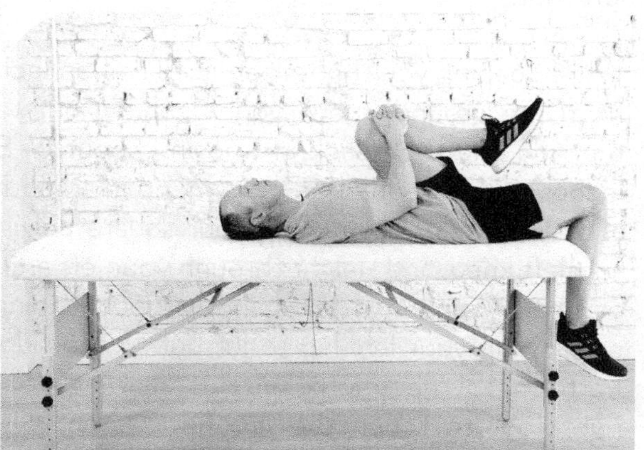

Hold your opposite knee close to your chest to protect your back and pelvis.

Standing Hip Strengthening

Note: If you have difficulty balancing, initially perform this exercise without an exercise tube and lightly hold on to a stable surface.

Stand and place an exercise tube or resistance band under both feet, where your heels meet the arches of your feet. Holding the handles or ends of the band, bend your elbows about 80–90 degrees. Lift your right foot approximately half an inch off the ground. Slightly rotate your right knee outward while maintaining a square (neutral) pelvis and facing forward. Soften your left knee and make sure you are bearing weight through the arch or heel—not the toes—of your left foot.

While keeping your right foot lifted half an inch from the ground, move your right leg out to the side and then back in (moving about 6–8 inches). Make sure the movement is smooth and slow while maintaining your square pelvis, soft left knee, and weight through your left arch or heel. Maintain a tall spine without leaning or allowing your left hip to jut out to the side. Perform 15 repetitions without allowing your right foot to touch the ground. Switch legs. Perform three sets on each leg.

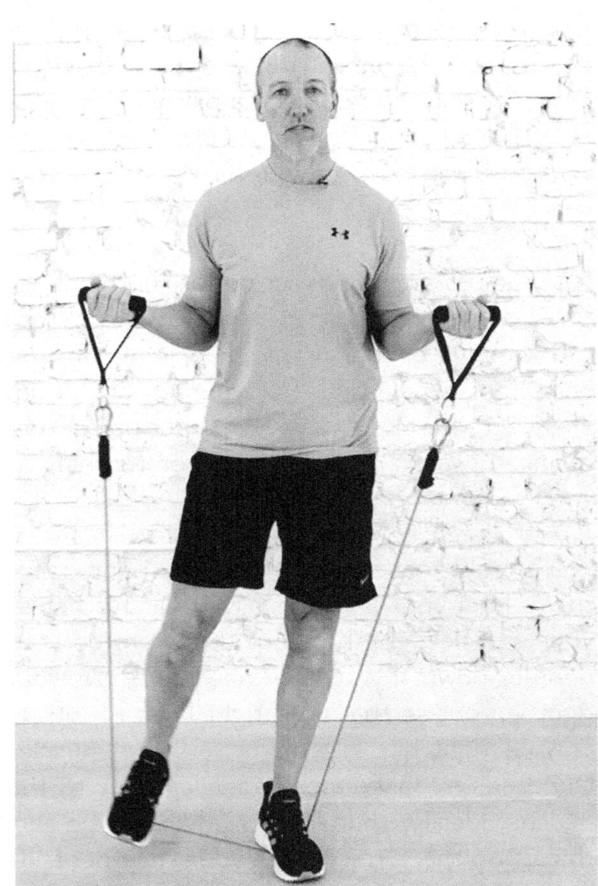

Maintain a soft stance knee and symmetrical upright posture during this exercise.

Butt Pumps

Assume a position on your elbows and knees with your lower spine flat, not sagging down toward the ground. Hold your lower spine in place by drawing in your belly button. Use your gluteals (butt muscles) to raise one leg in the air, with your knee bent 90 degrees. Stop at the point at which you feel the maximal contraction of your butt muscles. Do not overuse your low back or hamstring muscles to lift your leg.

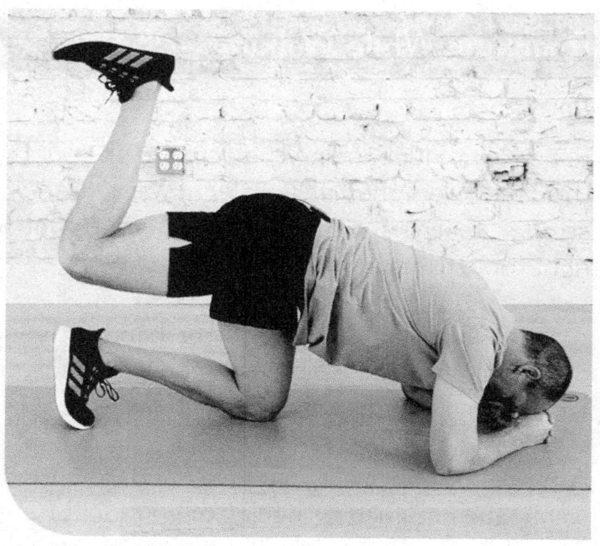

Perform a small pump of your leg up and down (about 1–2 inches) while maintaining the gluteal contraction. Do not lower your leg so far that you feel your gluteal muscles turn off; they should remain activated throughout the exercise. Perform 10–30 repetitions, until your gluteals fatigue. Be sure not to recruit your back or hamstring muscles when performing this exercise.

If you don't feel your butt muscles contracting, rotate your knee out slightly until you do, and then perform the pump. Switch sides. Perform two sets per session. Perform 2–3 times per day.

• • •

Videos are available for all exercises and habit changes presented in this book. Go to the website top3fix.com and enter your email and the code TOP3FIX to access them.

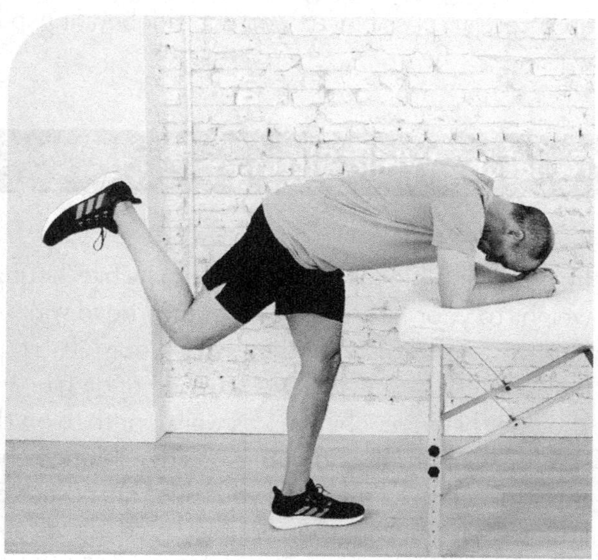

Gluteal strengthening is often the key to most lower body or back pain problems.

Fix Pain-Causing Habits

These exercises are designed to help fix dysfunctions in walking that lead to asymmetries and unilateral pain

Reaching While Walking

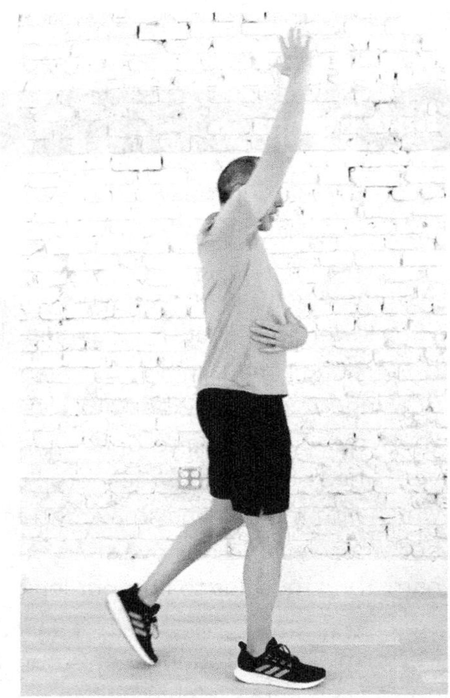

Learn to maintain a lengthened right waist while walking.

For a Right Sidebending Problem, reach your right arm up to the ceiling, lengthening your right waist. Walk with your right arm up, feeling the lengthening of your right waist at each right foot strike.

After 3–5 steps, rest your right hand on your head while continuing to walk, maintaining the length of your right waist and the engagement of your right gluteals.

After 3–5 steps, lower your right hand to your side, continuing to feel the natural lengthening of your right waist as you walk. Avoid hiking up your right shoulder to assist with this. Repeat as often as possible to correct sidebending patterns while walking.

Reaching While Sitting

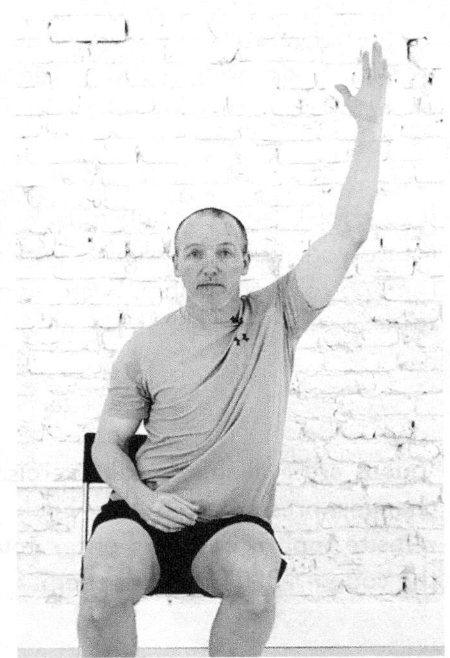

Learn to maintain a lengthened right waist while sitting.

For a Right Sidebending Problem, while sitting, shift your weight to your left hip and reach overhead with your left arm. Feel your left waist lengthen while your left hip pushes down into the chair seat relative to your right hip. Feel your left shoulder blade reaching up as well, lengthening the entire left side of your trunk and your shoulder. Notice that your right waist muscles contract and your right hip comes off the chair a little to help you lengthen your left side. Hold for two breaths.

Perform on the right side. Repeat on both sides, finishing with the right side to train your body to lengthen on the right side while sitting. Repeat frequently when sitting.

Gluteal Walking: Ice-Skating

Pretend you are ice-skating by taking a small lunge forward and slightly out to the side (like a hockey player) with your right leg, bending your knee and leaning forward slightly. Your weight should be mostly on your forward right leg. Pump twice up and down with your forward leg.

Place your hand on your right butt muscle and feel that it becomes firmer with this action. If your butt muscle does not become firmer, bend deeper at your knee and trunk until it does. Now step your left foot forward and repeat with your left leg. Continue for 10–20 steps, gradually straightening your trunk and forward leg until you reach an upright position, with your knee almost straight. You will likely notice that your butt muscles turn off at some point as you straighten up. Continue practicing until, with your trunk in a fully upright position, you feel natural gluteal activation when your forward foot strikes the ground.

Once in a tall, upright position, gradually return to a "normal"-looking walk but with your gluteal muscles activating naturally (not consciously) with each foot strike.

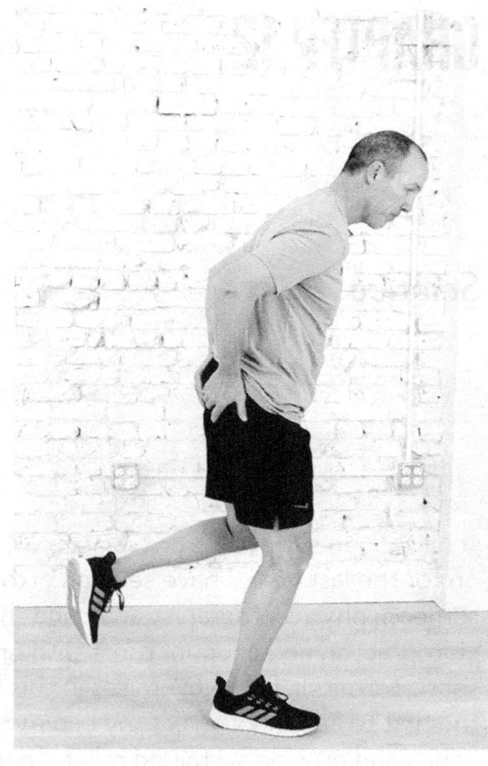

Mimicking ice-skating is a good way to activate your gluteal muscles to prepare for walking.

Gluteal Walking: Tiptoe Walking

Walk on your tiptoes for about 20 steps with your hands on your butt muscles. Feel that your butt muscles contract at each foot strike. This is not a conscious contraction but is instead one that occurs naturally. Then, slowly lower your heels back down and feel that your butt muscles continue to contract naturally as you take steps. Repeat throughout the day until, without needing to tiptoe walk first, you can walk with your gluteal muscles turning on naturally at each foot strike.

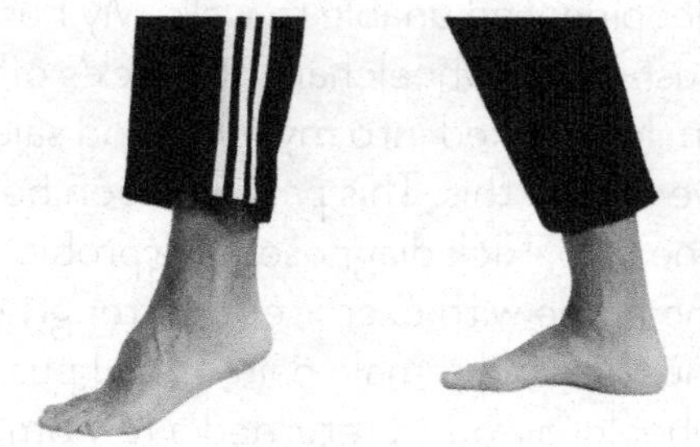

Tiptoe walking is a good way to activate your gluteal muscles to prepare for walking.

CHAPTER 12

Sciatica

"I have been suffering from sciatica off and on for the last year. I have seen an orthopedic surgeon, physical therapist, massage therapist, chiropractor, and acupuncturist with only short-term relief. The exercises in this book are the first to actually correct my bad movement habits and provide sustained relief. Thank you so much, Mr. Olderman!" **-Nathaniel C**

"I first met Rick Olderman several years ago. My doctor sent me to him because I had been suffering with sciatica for several weeks, not sleeping, and unable to walk. My husband pushed my wheelchair into Rick's office. Rick smiled, looked into my eyes, and said, 'Nancy, we can fix this. This pain will soon be gone.' In one visit, Rick diagnosed the problem and sent me home with exercises to strengthen weak muscles and remain pain-free. I pushed my wheelchair out! I returned a few times to make sure I was healing. The sciatica never returned." **-Nancy G**

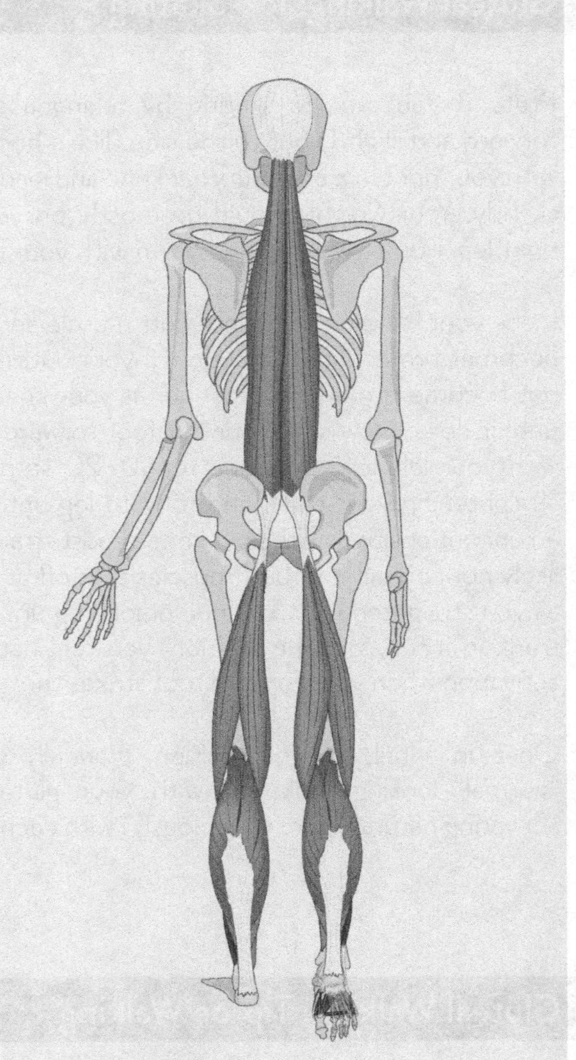

Pay special attention to asymmetries in strength, control, and range of motion. Your goals should include moving toward symmetry between the two legs.

Thigh Stretch

On a stable surface, such as a firm table or countertop, lie on your back with both knees drawn to your chest. Place a pillow under your head for additional comfort. Hold both knees with both hands to set your back and relax your legs.

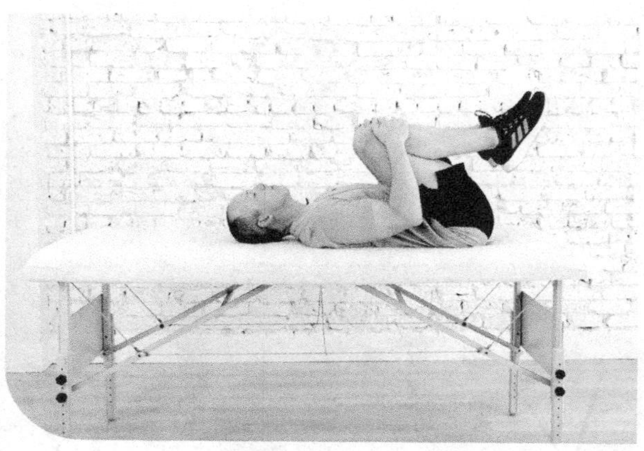

Hug both knees to your chest to set your back and pelvis.

Now, adjust your hands so they are both holding only your left knee. Slowly lower your right foot off the edge of the surface, keeping your right knee bent 90 degrees. Pull your left knee even closer to your chest to prevent your pelvis from rolling forward and your back from arching as you lower your right leg down.

You should feel a stretch in your right upper thigh. Feel your leg gradually lower further as your muscles lengthen, but do not force your right leg down. If you have knee pain, move your right leg out so that your right knee is outside of your right hip. Over time, as your muscles lengthen, gradually move your leg back to the midline. Ideally, your right thigh should be able to rest on the surface with your knee bent 90 degrees and positioned in line with your hip and shoulder. Hold for 7–10 breaths.

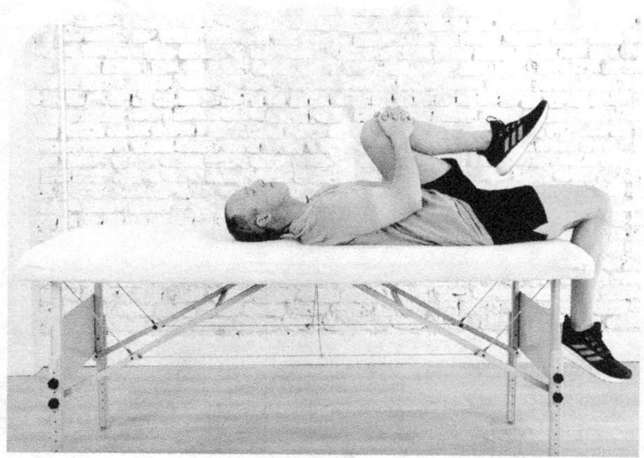

Hold your opposite knee close to your chest to protect your back and pelvis.

Bring your right leg back up to your chest and hug both knees to reset your back and pelvis. Repeat on the left side. Perform twice per side. Repeat 2–3 times per day.

Standing Hip Strengthening

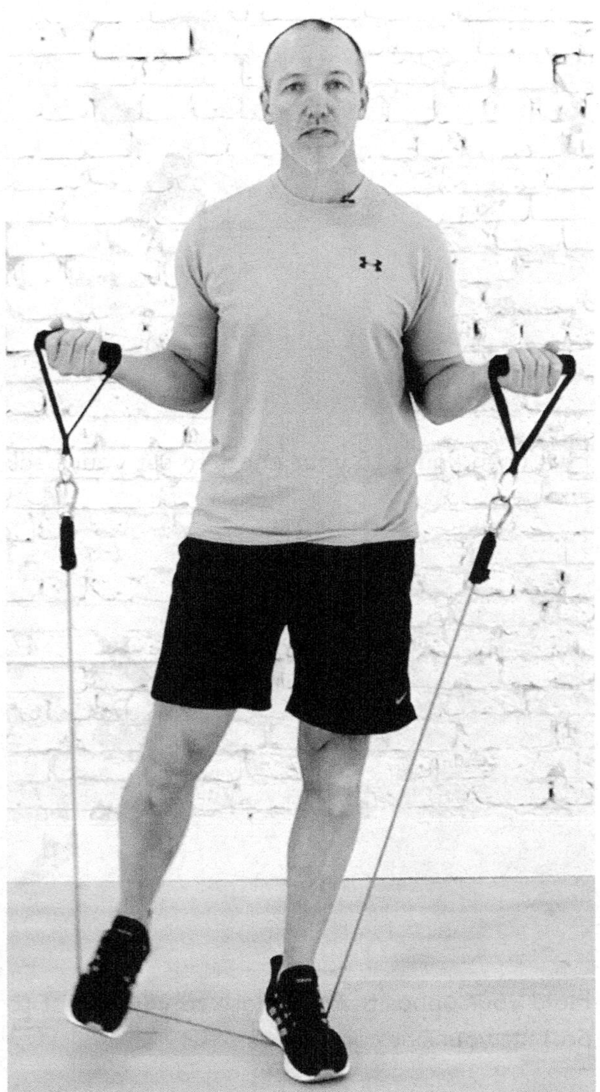

Maintain a soft stance knee and symmetrical upright posture during this exercise.

Note: If you have difficulty balancing, initially perform this exercise without an exercise tube and lightly hold on to a stable surface.

Stand and place an exercise tube or resistance band under both feet where your heels meet the arches of your feet. Holding the handles or ends of the band, bend your elbows about 80–90 degrees. Lift your right foot approximately half an inch off the ground. Slightly rotate your right knee outward while maintaining a square (neutral) pelvis and facing forward. Soften your left knee and make sure you are bearing weight through the arch or heel—not the toes—of your left foot.

While keeping your right foot lifted half an inch from the ground, move your right leg out to the side and then back in (moving about 6–8 inches). Make sure the movement is smooth and slow while maintaining your square pelvis, soft left knee, and weight through your left arch or heel. Maintain a tall spine without leaning or allowing your left hip to jut out to the side. Perform 15 repetitions without allowing your right foot to touch the ground. Switch legs. Perform three sets on each leg.

Butt Pumps

Assume a position on your elbows and knees with your lower spine flat, not sagging down toward the ground. Hold your lower spine in place by drawing in your belly button. Use your gluteals (butt muscles) to raise one leg in the air with your knee bent 90 degrees. Stop at the point at which you feel the maximal contraction of your butt muscles. Do not overuse your low back or hamstring muscles to lift your leg.

Perform a small pump of your leg up and down (about 1–2 inches) while maintaining the gluteal contraction. Do not lower your leg so far that you feel your gluteal muscles turn off; they should remain activated throughout the exercise. Perform 10–30 repetitions, until your gluteals fatigue. Be sure not to recruit your back or hamstring muscles when performing this exercise.

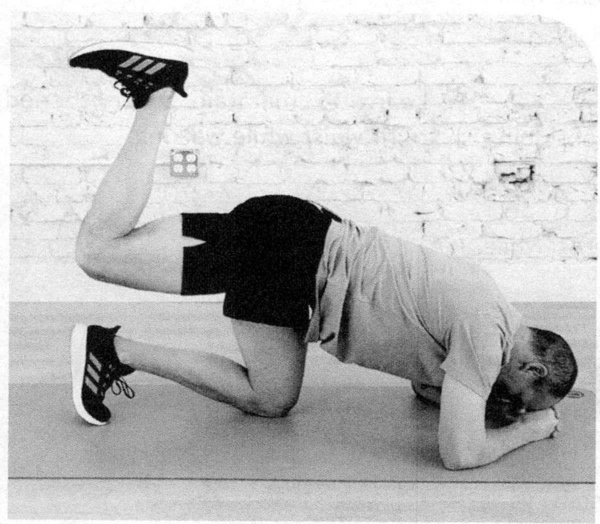

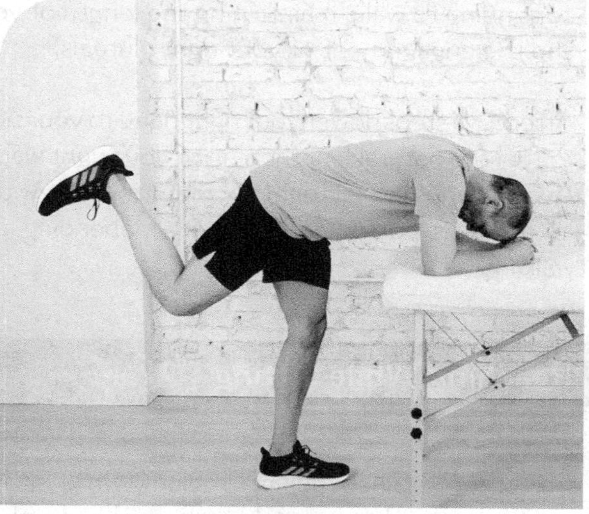

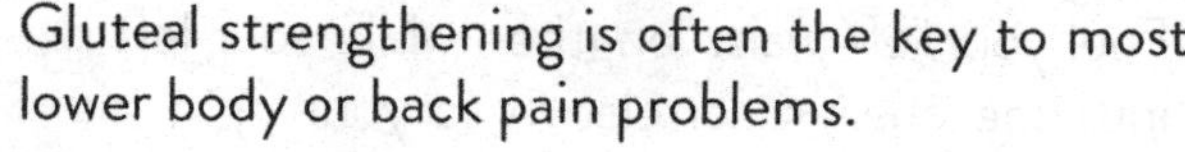

Gluteal strengthening is often the key to most lower body or back pain problems.

If you don't feel your butt muscles contracting, rotate your knee out slightly until you do, and then perform the pump. Switch sides. Perform two sets per session. Perform 2–3 times per day.

• • •

Videos are available for all exercises and habit changes presented in this book. Go to the website top3fix.com and enter your email and the code TOP3FIX to access them.

Fix Pain-Causing Habits

These exercises are designed to help fix dysfunctions in walking that lead to asymmetries and unilateral pain.

Reaching While Walking

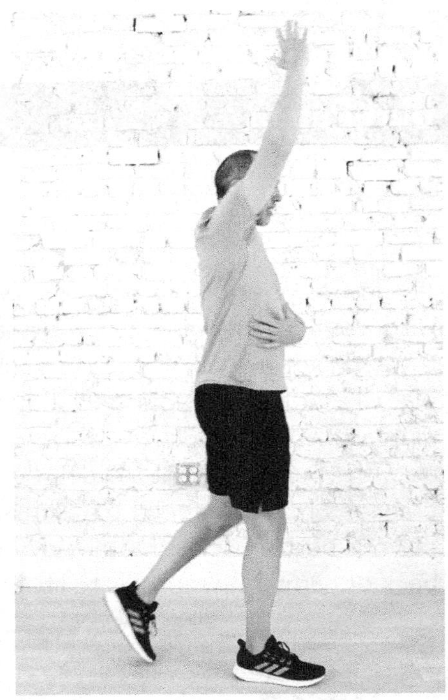

Learn to maintain a lengthened right waist while walking.

For a Right Sidebending Problem, reach your right arm up to the ceiling, lengthening your right waist. Walk with your right arm up, feeling the lengthening of your right waist at each right foot strike.

After 3–5 steps, rest your right hand on your head while continuing to walk, maintaining the length of your right waist and the engagement of your right gluteals.

After 3–5 steps, lower your right hand to your side, continuing to feel the natural lengthening of your right waist as you walk. Avoid hiking up your right shoulder to assist with this. Repeat as often as possible to correct sidebending patterns while walking.

Reaching While Sitting

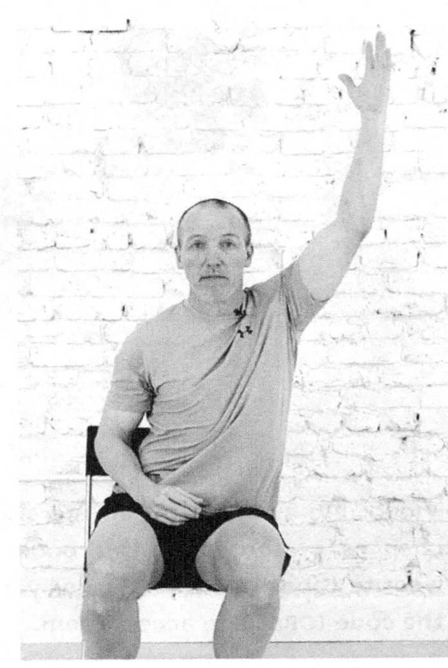

Learn to maintain a lengthened right waist while sitting.

For a Right Sidebending Problem, while sitting, shift your weight to your left hip and reach overhead with your left arm. Feel your left waist lengthen while your left hip pushes down into the chair seat relative to your right hip. Feel your left shoulder blade reaching up as well, lengthening the entire left side of your trunk and your shoulder. Notice that your right waist muscles contract and your right hip comes off the chair a little to help you lengthen your left side. Hold for two breaths.

Perform on the right side. Repeat on both sides, finishing with the right side to train your body to lengthen on the right side while sitting. Repeat frequently when sitting.

Gluteal Walking: Ice-Skating

Pretend you are ice-skating by taking a small lunge forward and slightly out to the side (like a hockey player) with your right leg, bending your knee and leaning forward slightly. Your weight should be mostly on your forward right leg. Pump twice up and down with your forward leg.

Place your hand on your right butt muscle and feel that it becomes firmer with this action. If your butt muscle does not become firmer, bend deeper at your knee and trunk until it does. Now step your left foot forward and repeat with your left leg. Continue for 10–20 steps, gradually straightening your trunk and forward leg until you reach an upright position, with your knee almost straight. You will likely notice that your butt muscles turn off at some point as you straighten up. Continue practicing until, with your trunk in a fully upright position, you feel natural gluteal activation when your forward foot strikes the ground.

Once in a tall, upright position, gradually return to a "normal"-looking walk but with your gluteal muscles activating naturally (not consciously) with each foot strike.

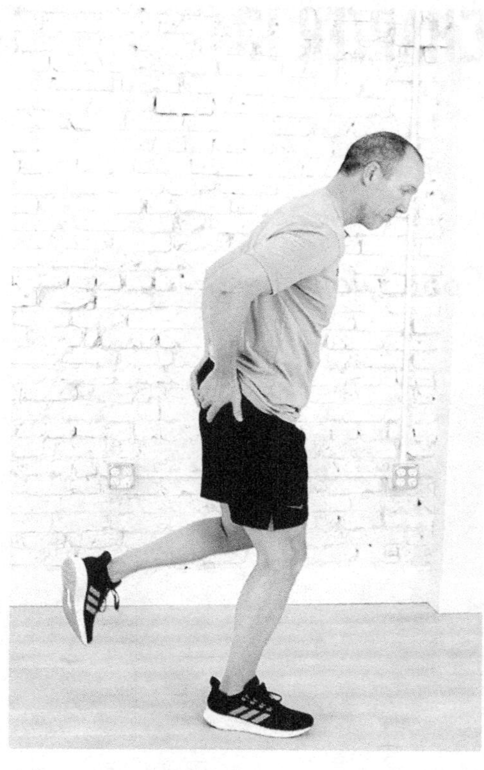

Mimicking ice-skating is a good way to activate your gluteal muscles to prepare for walking.

Gluteal Walking: Tiptoe Walking

Walk on your tiptoes for about 20 steps with your hands on your butt muscles. Feel that your butt muscles contract at each foot strike. This is not a conscious contraction but is instead one that occurs naturally. Then, slowly lower your heels back down and feel that your butt muscles continue to contract naturally as you take steps. Repeat throughout the day until, without needing to tiptoe walk first, you can walk with your gluteal muscles turning on naturally at each foot strike.

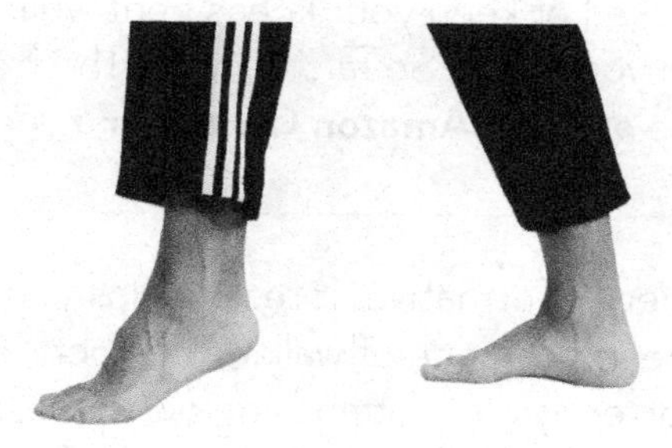

Tiptoe walking is a good way to activate your gluteal muscles to prepare for walking.

CHAPTER 13

Spondylolisthesis

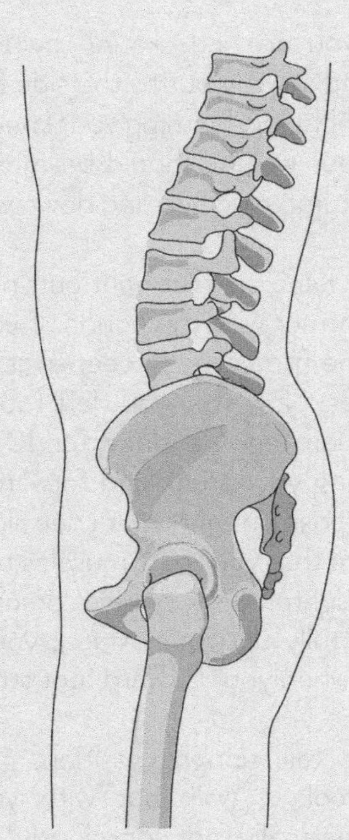

"In the first 48 hours, I was pretty sure this was going to help my four-year-long problem. No one has ever said don't stand with your knees locked or keep your knees bent while lying flat on your back. So far, so good. The free videos are great!" **-Amazon Customer**

"Very informative. It really helps you to see the importance of walking correctly, sitting correctly and not abusing our spines. The exercises really help." **-Amazon Customer**

Spondylolisthesis is an Extension Problem. The focus of these exercises is to reduce the forces pulling the spine into a more arched, or extended, position. Pay special attention to asymmetries in strength, control, and range of motion. Your goals should include moving toward symmetry between the two legs.

Thigh Stretch

On a stable surface, such as a firm table or countertop, lie on your back with both knees drawn to your chest. Place a pillow under your head for additional comfort. Hold both knees with both hands to set your back and relax your legs.

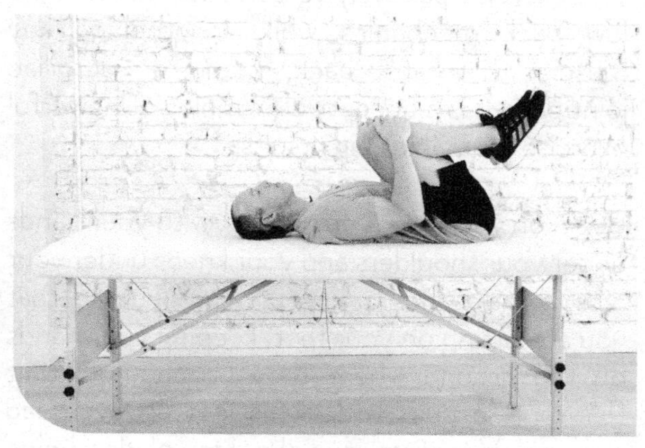

Hug both knees to your chest to set your back and pelvis.

Now, adjust your hands so they are both holding only your left knee. Slowly lower your right foot off the edge of the surface, keeping your right knee bent 90 degrees. Pull your left knee even closer to your chest to prevent your pelvis from rolling forward and your back from arching as you lower your right leg down.

You should feel a stretch in your right upper thigh. Feel your leg gradually lower further as your muscles lengthen, but do not force your right leg down. If you have knee pain, move your right leg out so that your right knee is outside of your right hip. Over time, as your muscles lengthen, gradually move your leg back to the midline. Ideally, your right thigh should be able to rest on the surface with your knee bent 90 degrees and positioned in line with your hip and shoulder. Hold for 7–10 breaths.

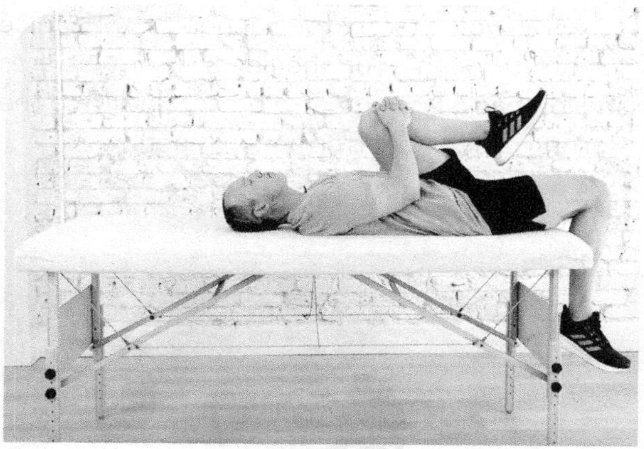

Hold your opposite knee close to your chest to protect your back and pelvis.

Bring your right leg back up to your chest and hug both knees to reset your back and pelvis. Repeat on the left side. Perform twice per side. Repeat 2–3 times per day.

All-Fours Rocking Stretch

This exercise passively restores normal hip and low back mechanics while lengthening key muscles that cause back, sciatic, or sacroiliac joint pain. It is a deceptively simple yet powerful exercise that yields big results.

Begin on your hands and knees, with your hands under your shoulders and your knees under your hips. Exhale and rock your hips back so that you are sitting on your feet, keeping your hands on the ground where they began. Feel that this motion pulls your arms into an overhead position. Visualize your shoulder blades being pulled up toward the top of your head. Slide your hands forward, if you are able, to accentuate this stretch. Feel free to rest your head on a small pillow, if you prefer, for support. Feel a nice stretch through your shoulders or armpit area and low back. Breathe 3–5 times. Return to the starting position. Perform 3–5 repetitions.

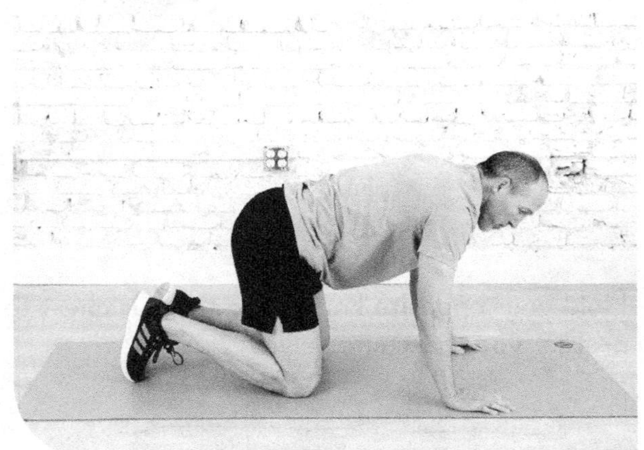

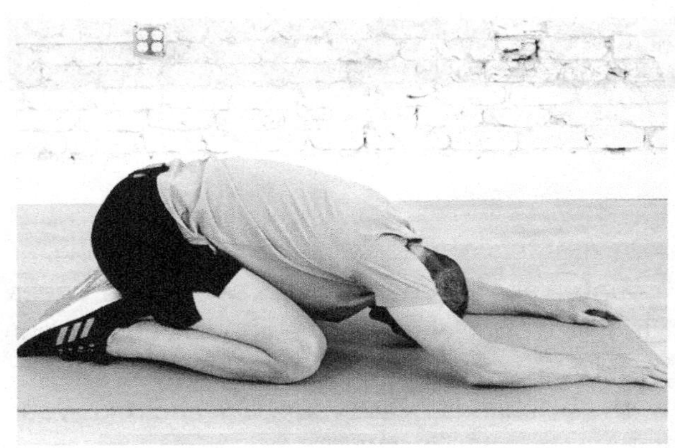

You should feel a stretch in your shoulders, chest, or arms during this exercise.

Take this stretch up a notch after sitting back on your heels by walking both hands to the left. Take three breaths and then walk your hands to the right. If your neck, shoulder, or headache pain is on one side, for example the right side, you'll likely find that your right shoulder and rib cage feel tighter. Solving that tightness will help solve your pain.

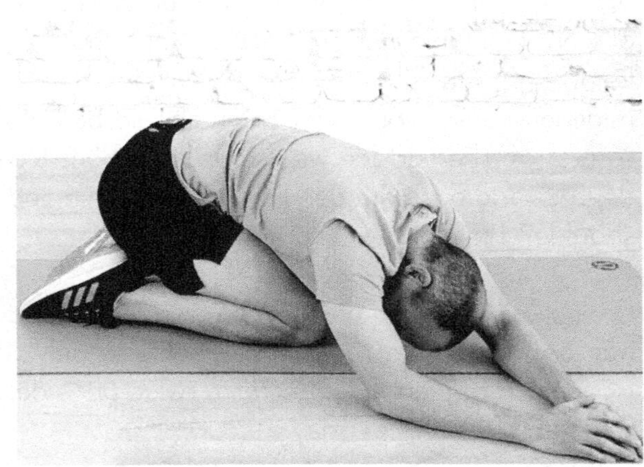

Sidebending while stretching can help you solve unilateral tightness contributing to your pain.

Butt Pumps

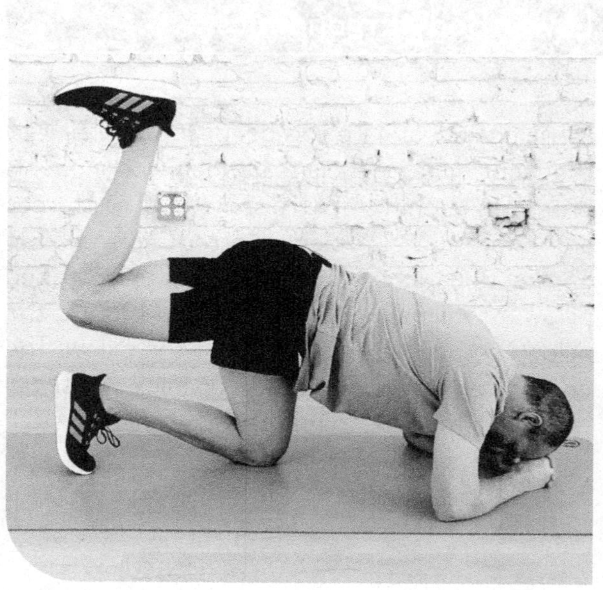

Assume a position on your elbows and knees with your lower spine flat, not sagging down toward the ground. Hold your lower spine in place by drawing in your belly button. Use your gluteals (butt muscles) to raise one leg in the air with your knee bent 90 degrees. Stop at the point at which you feel the maximal contraction of your butt muscles. Do not overuse your low back or hamstring muscles to lift your leg.

Perform a small pump of your leg up and down (about 1–2 inches) while maintaining the gluteal contraction. Do not lower your leg so far that you feel your gluteal muscles turn off; they should remain activated throughout the exercise. Perform 10–30 repetitions, until your gluteals fatigue. Be sure not to recruit your back or hamstring muscles when performing this exercise.

If you don't feel your butt muscles contracting, rotate your knee out slightly until you do, and then perform the pump. Switch sides. Perform two sets per session. Perform 2–3 times per day.

• • •

Videos are available for all exercises and habit changes presented in this book. Go to the website top3fix.com and enter your email and the code TOP3FIX to access them.

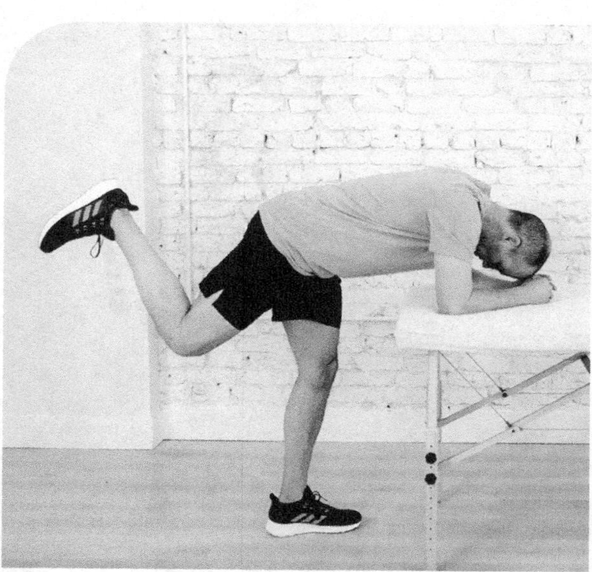

Gluteal strengthening is often the key to most lower body or back pain problems.

Fix Pain-Causing Habits

Lower Body Ergonomics

Most chair seats are too deep, so people sit at the front edge of their seat when working. This promotes arching of the spine and reinforces an Extension Problem pattern of muscle contraction. To solve this, simply place a bed pillow or two behind your back. Orient the pillows vertically. Lean back into the pillow. The contact of the pillow with your back will signal your back muscles to relax.

Additionally, place a box under your feet to raise your knees higher than your hip joints. This will gently roll your pelvis back, flattening your spine.

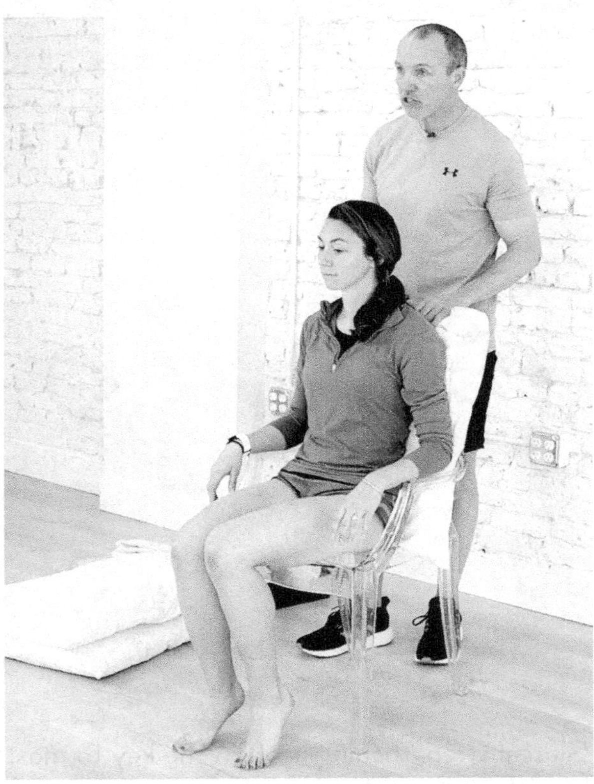

Placing pillows in the back of your chair will signal your back muscles to relax.

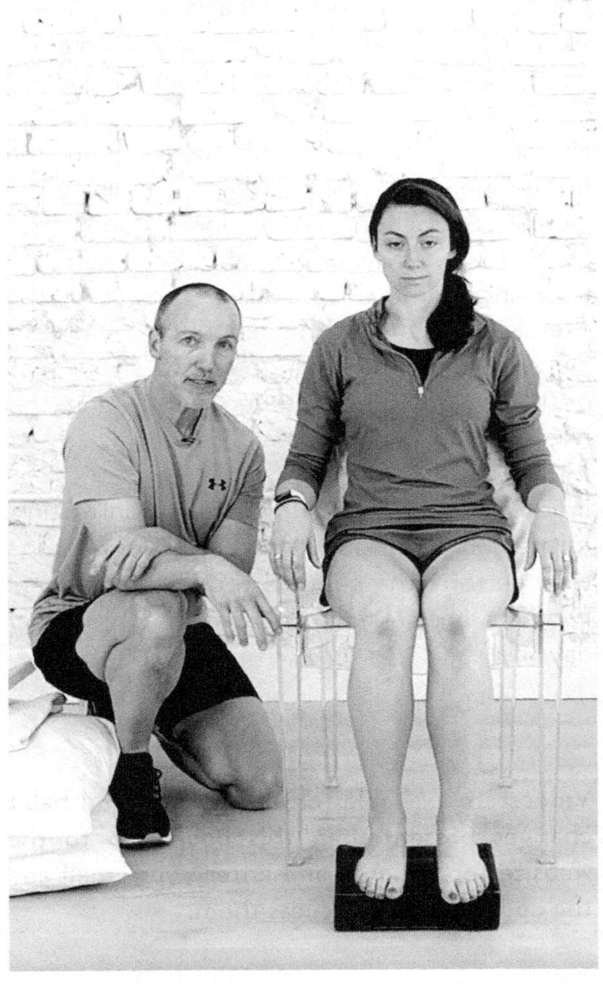

Adding support under your feet helps to tilt your pelvis back and flatten your spine.

Gluteal Walking: Ice-Skating

Pretend you are ice-skating by taking a small lunge forward and slightly out to the side (like a hockey player) with your right leg, bending your knee and leaning forward slightly. Your weight should be mostly on your forward right leg. Pump twice up and down with your forward leg.

Place your hand on your right butt muscle and feel that it becomes firmer with this action. If your butt muscle does not become firmer, bend deeper at your knee and trunk until it does. Now step your left foot forward and repeat with your left leg. Continue for 10–20 steps, gradually straightening your trunk and forward leg until you reach an upright position, with your knee almost straight. You will likely notice that your butt muscles turn off at some point as you straighten up. Continue practicing until, with your trunk in a fully upright position, you feel natural gluteal activation when your forward foot strikes the ground.

Once in a tall, upright position, gradually return to a "normal"-looking walk but with your gluteal muscles activating naturally (not consciously) with each foot strike.

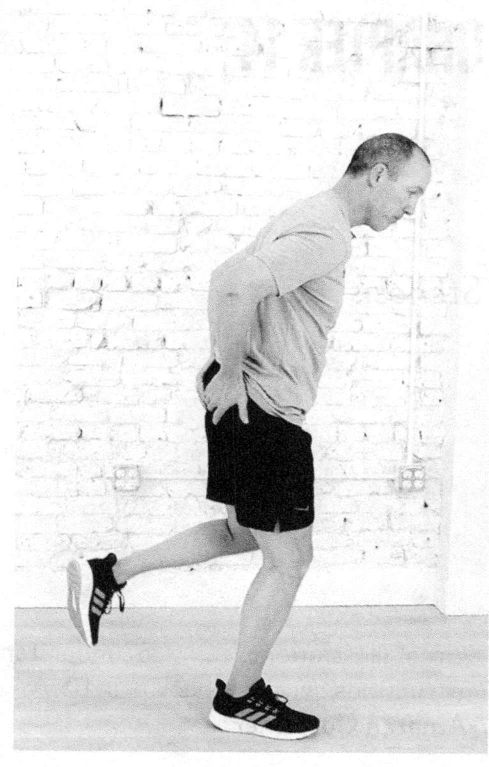

Mimicking ice-skating is a good way to activate your gluteal muscles to prepare for walking.

Gluteal Walking: Tiptoe Walking

Walk on your tiptoes for about 20 steps with your hands on your butt muscles. Feel that your butt muscles contract at each foot strike. This is not a conscious contraction but is instead one that occurs naturally. Then, slowly lower your heels back down and feel that your butt muscles continue to contract naturally as you take steps. Repeat throughout the day until, without needing to tiptoe walk first, you can walk with your gluteal muscles turning on naturally at each foot strike.

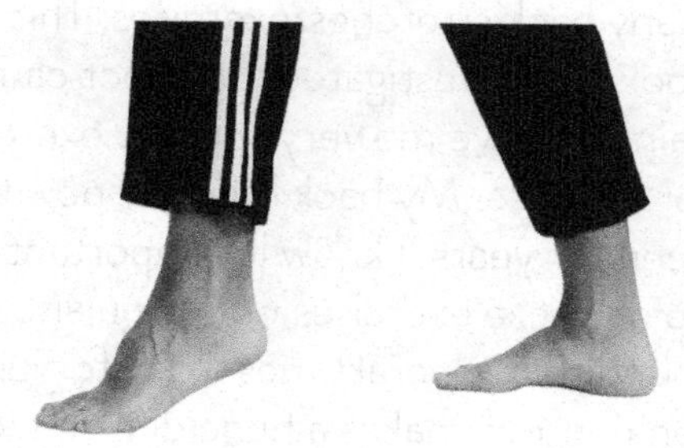

Tiptoe walking is a good way to activate your gluteal muscles to prepare for walking.

CHAPTER 14

Stenosis

"Great illustrations, easy-to-understand instructions. My best back pain book."
-Amazon Customer

"I got this book at the library but liked it so much that I will now order it from Amazon. I am 70 years old and have had back pain for 15 years. I have tried numerous ways to deal with it, including chiropractic, massage, Pilates, and many back stretches/exercises. This is the first book that investigated the exact causes of my pain and gave me very specific exercises to do for my case. My back is better now than it has been for years. I know it's important to keep doing these exercises on a regular basis. I have found that several times a day for just five or ten minutes makes a huge difference. I really appreciate the videos that correspond with this book." **-Amazon Customer**

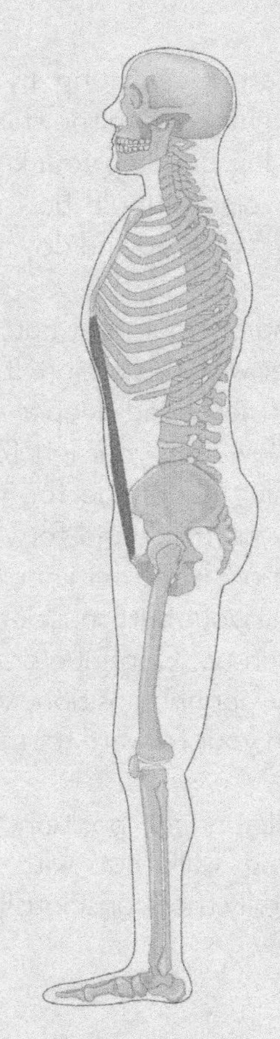

Stenosis is an Extension Problem. The focus of these exercises is to reduce the forces pulling the spine into a more arched, or extended, position. Pay special attention to asymmetries in strength, control, and range of motion. Your goals should include moving toward symmetry between the two legs.

Thigh Stretch

On a stable surface, such as a firm table or countertop, lie on your back with both knees drawn to your chest. Place a pillow under your head for additional comfort. Hold both knees with both hands to set your back and relax your legs.

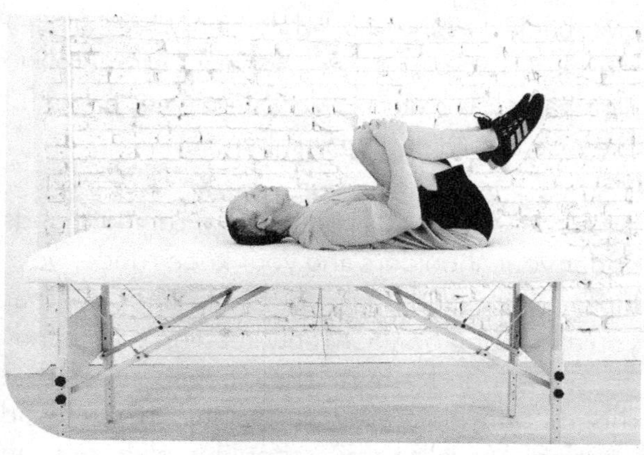

Hug both knees to your chest to set your back and pelvis.

Now, adjust your hands so they are both holding only your left knee. Slowly lower your right foot off the edge of the surface, keeping your right knee bent 90 degrees. Pull your left knee even closer to your chest to prevent your pelvis from rolling forward and your back from arching as you lower your right leg down.

You should feel a stretch in your right upper thigh. Feel your leg gradually lower further as your muscles lengthen, but do not force your right leg down. If you have knee pain, move your right leg out so that your right knee is outside of your right hip. Over time, as your muscles lengthen, gradually move your leg back to midline. Ideally, your right thigh should be able to rest on the surface with your knee bent 90 degrees and positioned in line with your hip and shoulder. Hold for 7–10 breaths.

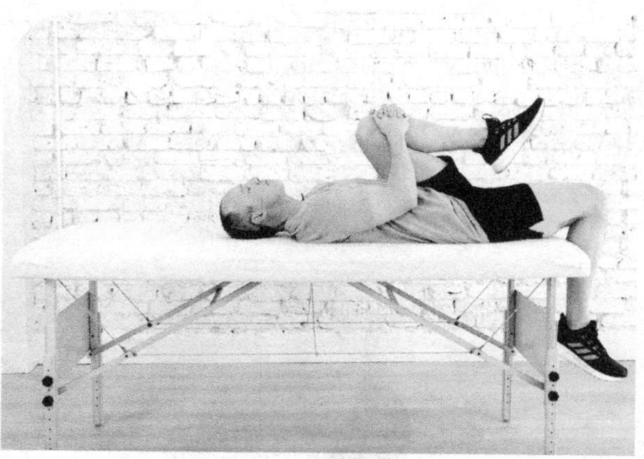

Hold your opposite knee close to your chest to protect your back and pelvis.

Bring your right leg back up to your chest and hug both knees to reset your back and pelvis. Repeat on the left side. Perform twice per side. Repeat 2–3 times per day.

All-Fours Rocking Stretch

This exercise passively restores normal hip and low back mechanics while lengthening key muscles that cause back, sciatic, or sacroiliac joint pain. It is a deceptively simple yet powerful exercise that yields big results.

Begin on your hands and knees with your hands under your shoulders and your knees under your hips. Exhale and rock your hips back so that you are sitting on your feet, keeping your hands on the ground where they began. Feel that this motion pulls your arms into an overhead position. Visualize your shoulder blades being pulled up toward the top of your head. Slide your hands forward, if you are able, to accentuate this stretch. Feel free to rest your head on a small pillow, if you prefer, for support. Feel a nice stretch through your shoulders or armpit area and low back. Breathe 3–5 times. Return to the starting position. Perform 3–5 repetitions.

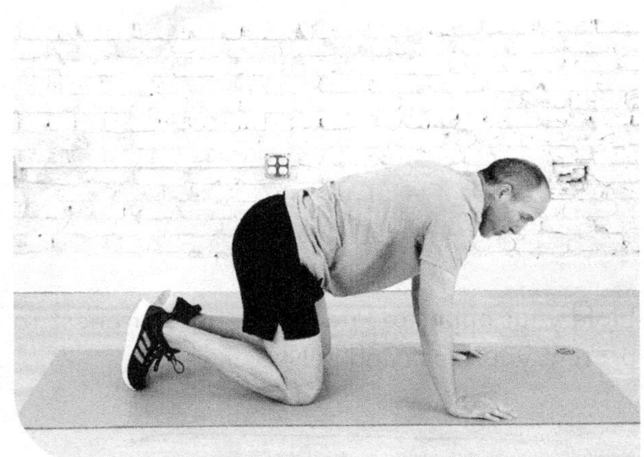

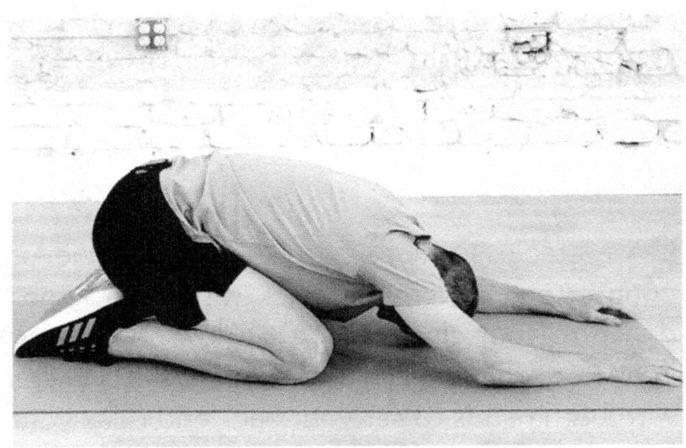

You should feel a stretch in your shoulders, chest, or arms during this exercise.

Take this stretch up a notch after sitting back on your heels by walking both hands to the left. Take three breaths and then walk your hands to the right. If your neck, shoulder, or headache pain is on one side, for example the right side, you'll likely find that your right shoulder and rib cage feel tighter. Solving that tightness will help solve your pain.

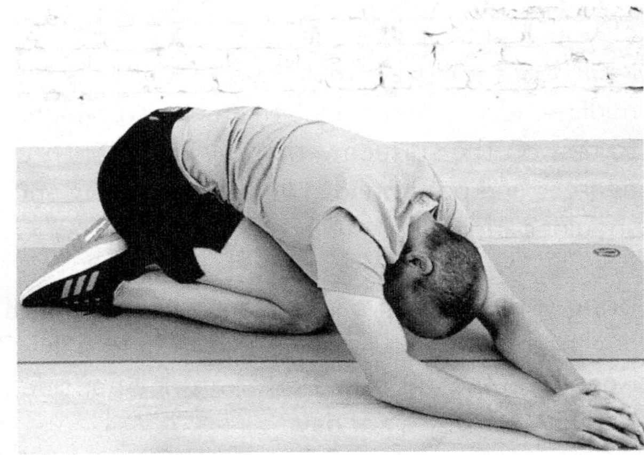

Sidebending while stretching can help you solve unilateral tightness contributing to your pain.

Butt Pumps

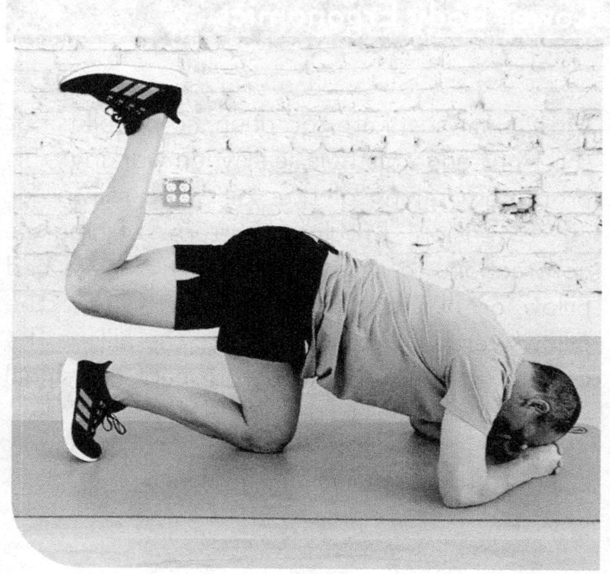

Assume a position on your elbows and knees with your lower spine flat, not sagging down toward the ground. Hold your lower spine in place by drawing in your belly button. Use your gluteals (butt muscles) to raise one leg in the air with your knee bent 90 degrees. Stop at the point at which you feel the maximal contraction of your butt muscles. Do not overuse your low back or hamstring muscles to lift your leg.

Perform a small pump of your leg up and down (about 1–2 inches) while maintaining the gluteal contraction. Do not lower your leg so far that you feel your gluteal muscles turn off; they should remain activated throughout the exercise. Perform 10–30 repetitions, until your gluteals fatigue. Be sure not to recruit your back or hamstring muscles when performing this exercise.

If you don't feel your butt muscles contracting, rotate your knee out slightly until you do, and then perform the pump. Switch sides. Perform twice per session. Perform 2–3 times per day.

• • •

Videos are available for all exercises and habit changes presented in this book. Go to the website top3fix.com and enter your email and the code TOP3FIX to access them.

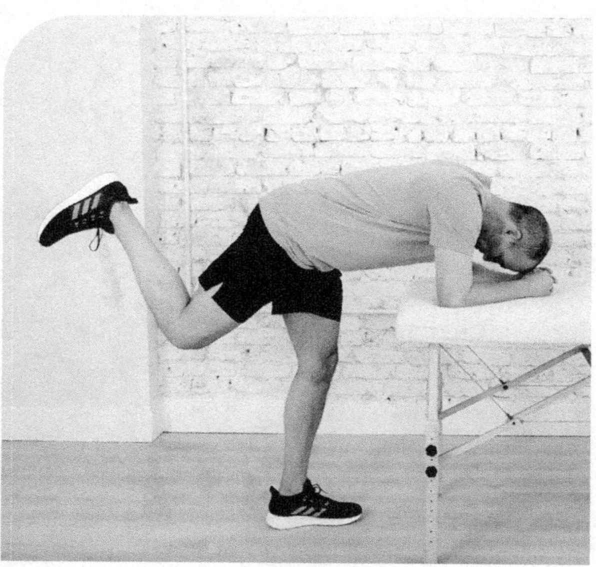

Gluteal strengthening is often the key to most lower body or back pain problems.

Fix Pain-Causing Habits

Lower Body Ergonomics

Most chair seats are too deep, so people sit at the front edge of their seat when working. This promotes arching of the spine and reinforces an Extension Problem pattern of muscle contraction. To solve this, simply place a bed pillow or two behind your back. Orient the pillows vertically. Lean back into the pillow. The contact of the pillow with your back will signal your back muscles to relax.

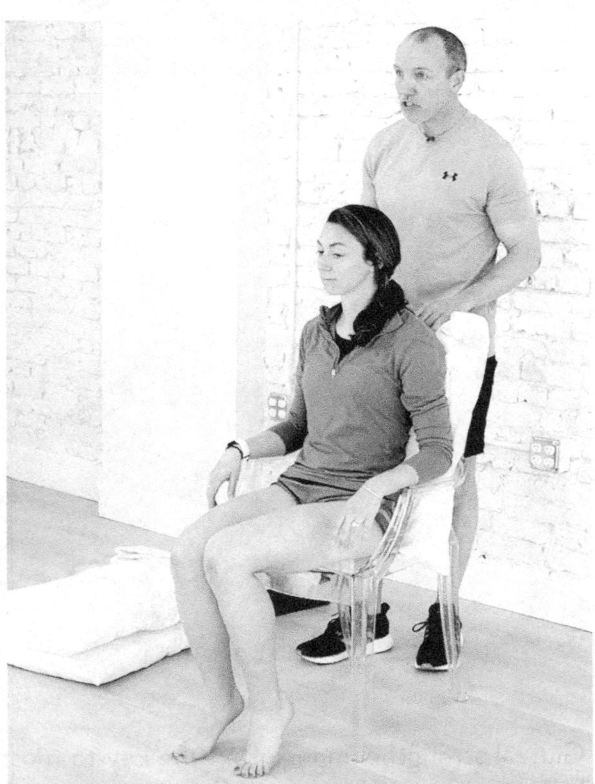

Placing pillows in the back of your chair will signal your back muscles to relax.

Additionally, place a box under your feet to raise your knees higher than your hip joints. This will gently roll your pelvis back, flattening your spine.

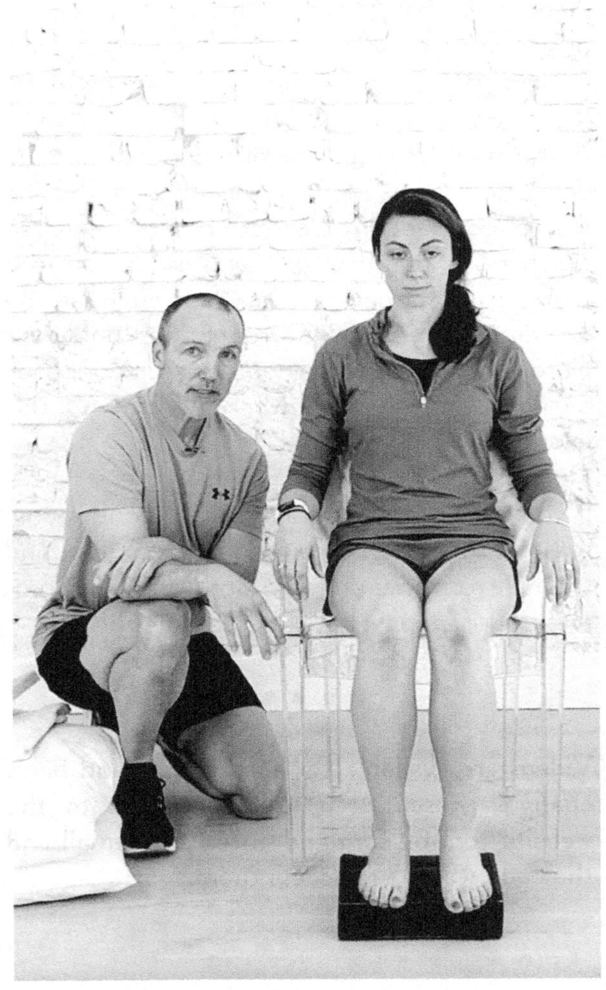

Adding support under your feet helps to tilt your pelvis back and flatten your spine.

Gluteal Walking: Ice-Skating

Pretend you are ice-skating by taking a small lunge forward and slightly out to the side (like a hockey player) with your right leg, bending your knee and leaning forward slightly. Your weight should be mostly on your forward right leg. Pump twice up and down with your forward leg.

Place your hand on your right butt muscle and feel that it becomes firmer with this action. If your butt muscle does not become firmer, bend deeper at your knee and trunk until it does. Now step your left foot forward and repeat with your left leg. Continue for 10–20 steps, gradually straightening your trunk and forward leg until you reach an upright position, with your knee almost straight. You will likely notice that your butt muscles turn off at some point as you straighten up. Continue practicing until, with your trunk in a fully upright position, you feel natural gluteal activation when your forward foot strikes the ground.

Once in a tall, upright position, gradually return to a "normal"-looking walk but with your gluteal muscles activating naturally (not consciously) with each foot strike.

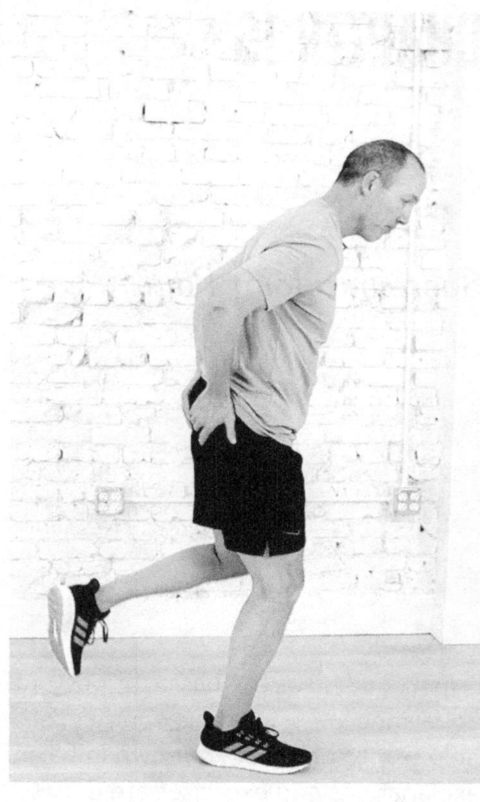

Mimicking ice-skating is a good way to activate your gluteal muscles to prepare for walking.

Gluteal Walking: Tiptoe Walking

Walk on your tiptoes for about 20 steps with your hands on your butt muscles. Feel that your butt muscles contract at each foot strike. This is not a conscious contraction but is instead one that occurs naturally. Then, slowly lower your heels back down and feel that your butt muscles continue to contract naturally as you take steps. Repeat throughout the day until, without needing to tiptoe walk first, you can walk with your gluteal muscles turning on naturally at each foot strike.

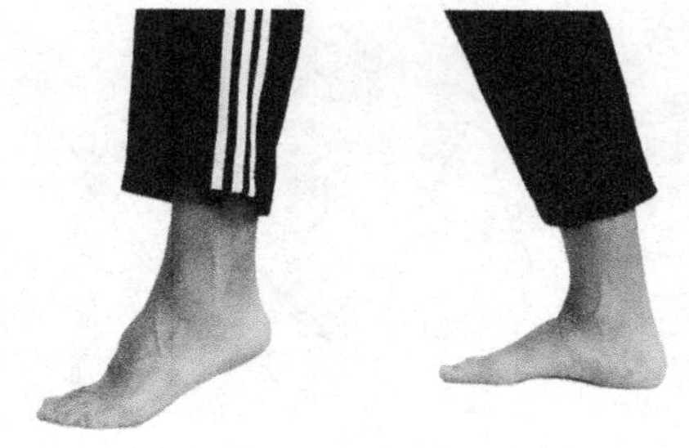

Tiptoe walking is a good way to activate your gluteal muscles to prepare for walking.

CHAPTER 15

Sacroiliac Joint Pain

"Rick condenses the basics of postural imbalance in easy-to-recognize exercises that help you to uncover your own imbalances. The explanations and exercises are easy to follow to guide you to finding a solution to your chronic pain." **-Amazon Customer**

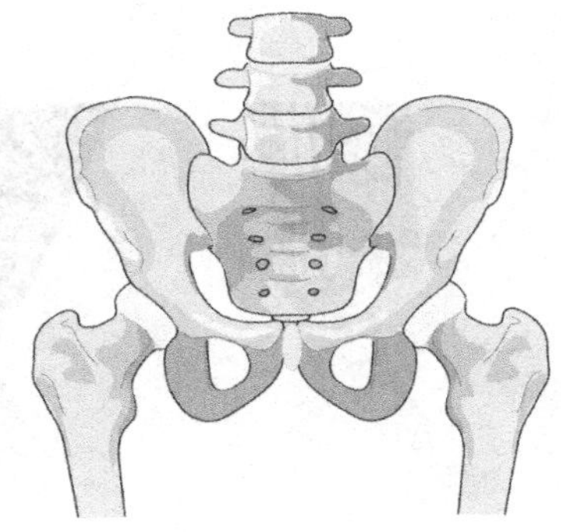

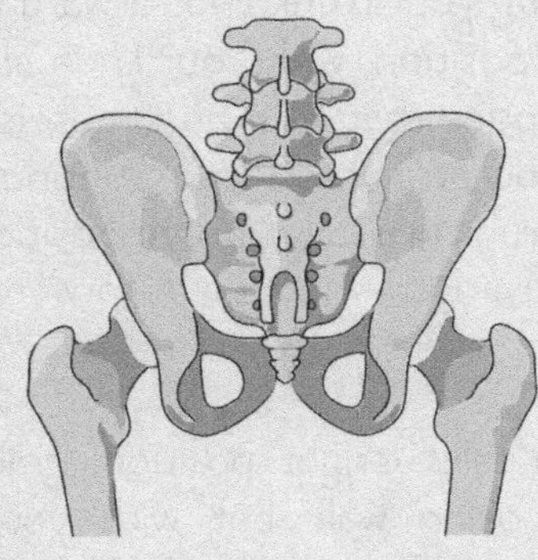

Sacroiliac joint pain typically occurs because of asymmetrical forces acting on the pelvis, which create sheer and torque across the sacroiliac joint. Pay special attention to asymmetries in strength, control, and range of motion. Your goals should include moving toward symmetry between the two legs.

Thigh Stretch

On a stable surface, such as a firm table or countertop, lie on your back with both knees drawn to your chest. Place a pillow under your head for additional comfort. Hold both knees with both hands to set your back and relax your legs.

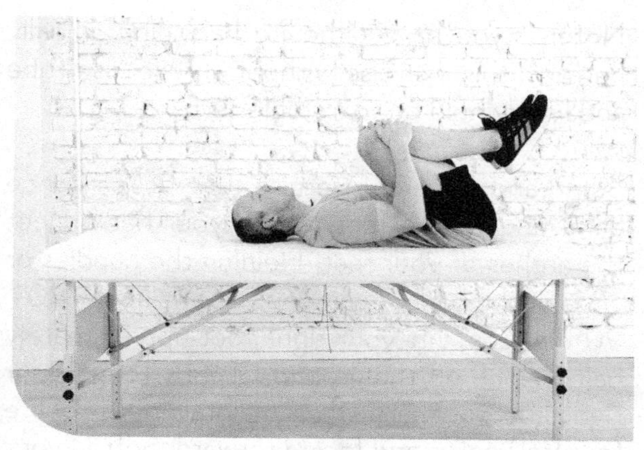

Hug both knees to your chest to set your back and pelvis.

Now, adjust your hands so they are both holding only your left knee. Slowly lower your right foot off the edge of the surface, keeping your right knee bent 90 degrees. Pull your left knee even closer to your chest to prevent your pelvis from rolling forward and your back from arching as you lower your right leg down.

You should feel a stretch in your right upper thigh. Feel your leg gradually lower further as your muscles lengthen, but do not force your right leg down. If you have knee pain, move your right leg out so that your right knee is outside of your right hip. Over time, as your muscles lengthen, gradually move your leg back to the midline. Ideally, your right thigh should be able to rest on the surface with your knee bent 90 degrees and positioned in line with your hip and shoulder. Hold for 7–10 breaths.

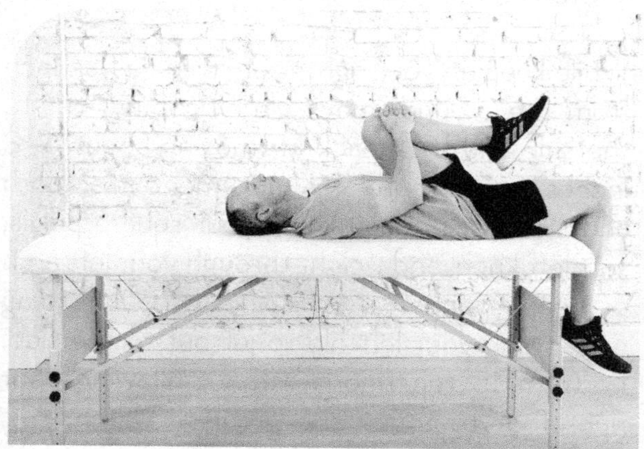

Hold your opposite knee close to your chest to protect your back and pelvis.

Bring your right leg back up to your chest and hug both knees to reset your back and pelvis. Repeat on the left side. Perform twice per side. Repeat 2–3 times per day.

Standing Hip Strengthening

Note: If you have difficulty balancing, initially perform this exercise without an exercise tube and lightly hold on to a stable surface.

Stand and place an exercise tube or resistance band under both feet, where your heels meet the arches of your feet. Holding the handles or ends of the band, bend your elbows about 80–90 degrees. Lift your right foot approximately half an inch off the ground. Slightly rotate your right knee outward while maintaining a square (neutral) pelvis and facing forward. Soften your left knee and make sure you are bearing weight through the arch or heel—not the toes—of your left foot.

While keeping your right foot lifted half an inch from the ground, move your right leg out to the side and then back in (moving about 6–8 inches). Make sure the movement is smooth and slow while maintaining your square pelvis, soft left knee, and weight through your left arch or heel. Maintain a tall spine without leaning or allowing your left hip to jut out to the side. Perform 15 repetitions without allowing your right foot to touch the ground. Switch legs. Perform three sets on each leg.

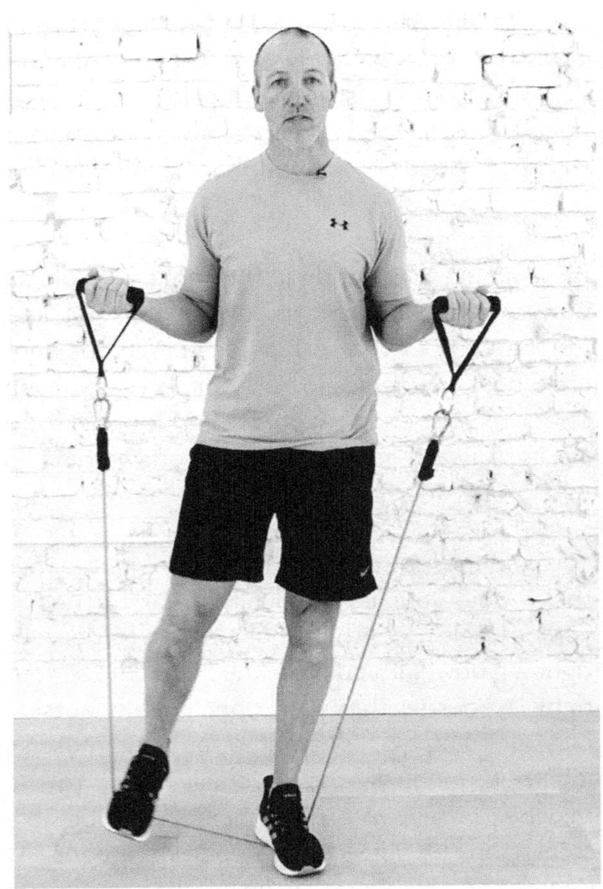

Maintain a soft stance knee and symmetrical upright posture during this exercise.

Butt Pumps

Assume a position on your elbows and knees with your lower spine flat, not sagging down toward the ground. Hold your lower spine in place by drawing in your belly button. Use your gluteals (butt muscles) to raise one leg in the air with your knee bent 90 degrees. Stop at the point at which you feel the maximal contraction of your butt muscles. Do not overuse your low back or hamstring muscles to lift your leg.

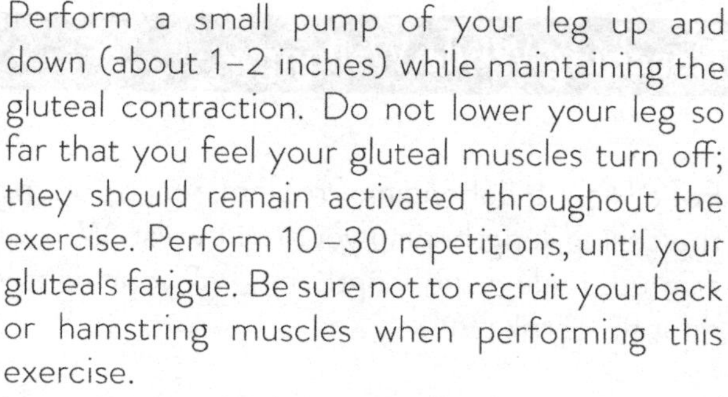

Perform a small pump of your leg up and down (about 1–2 inches) while maintaining the gluteal contraction. Do not lower your leg so far that you feel your gluteal muscles turn off; they should remain activated throughout the exercise. Perform 10–30 repetitions, until your gluteals fatigue. Be sure not to recruit your back or hamstring muscles when performing this exercise.

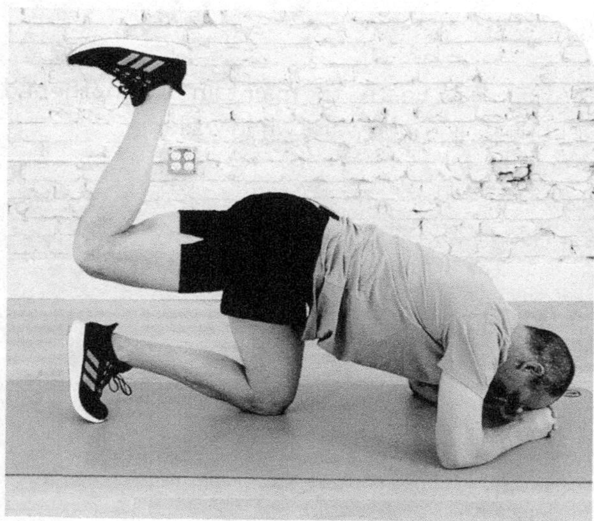

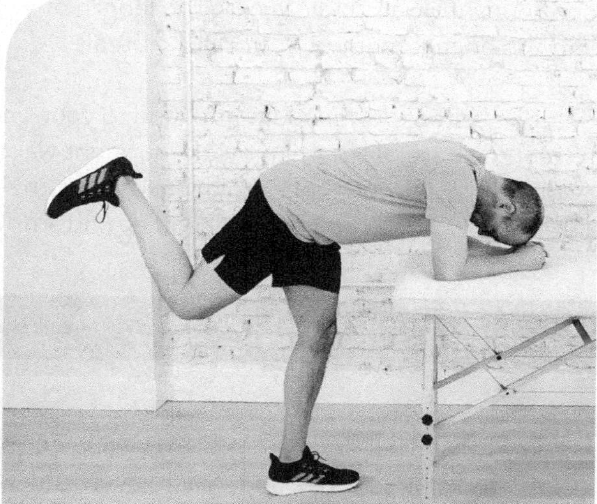

• • •

Videos are available for all exercises and habit changes presented in this book. Go to the website top3fix.com and enter your email and the code TOP3FIX to access them.

Gluteal strengthening is often the key to most lower body or back pain problems.

If you don't feel your butt muscles contracting, rotate your knee out slightly until you do, and then perform the pump. Switch sides. Perform two sets per session. Perform 2–3 times per day.

Fix Pain-Causing Habits

These exercises are designed to help fix dysfunctions in walking that lead to asymmetries and unilateral pain.

Reaching While Walking

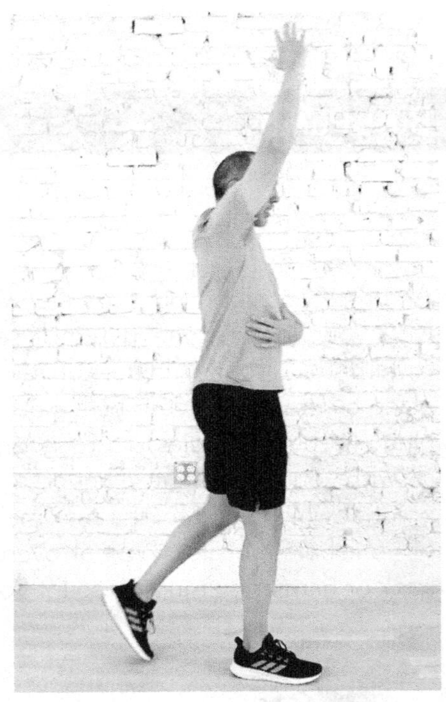

Learn to maintain a lengthened right waist while walking.

For a Right Sidebending Problem, reach your right arm up to the ceiling, lengthening your right waist. Walk with your right arm up, feeling the lengthening of your right waist at each right foot strike.

After 3–5 steps, rest your right hand on your head while continuing to walk, maintaining the length of your right waist and the engagement of your right gluteals.

After 3–5 steps, lower your right hand to your side, continuing to feel the natural lengthening of your right waist as you walk. Avoid hiking up your right shoulder to assist with this. Repeat as often as possible to correct sidebending patterns while walking.

Reaching While Sitting

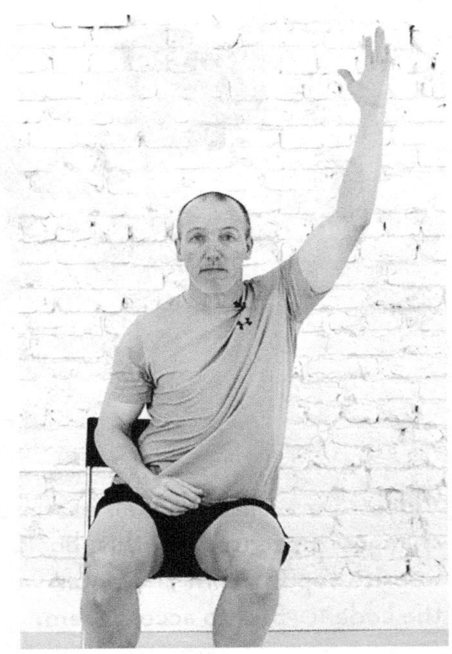

Learn to maintain a lengthened right waist while sitting.

For a Right Sidebending Problem, while sitting, shift your weight to your left hip and reach overhead with your left arm. Feel your left waist lengthen while your left hip pushes down into the chair seat relative to your right hip. Feel your left shoulder blade reaching up as well so the entire left side of your trunk and your shoulder have lengthened. Notice that your right waist muscles contract and your right hip comes off the chair a little to help you lengthen your left side. Hold for two breaths.

Perform on the right side. Repeat on both sides, finishing with the right side to train your body to lengthen on the right side while sitting. Repeat frequently when sitting.

Gluteal Walking: Ice-Skating

Pretend you are ice-skating by taking a small lunge forward and slightly out to the side (like a hockey player) with your right leg, bending your knee and leaning forward slightly. Your weight should be mostly on your forward right leg. Pump twice up and down with your forward leg.

Place your hand on your right butt muscle and feel that it becomes firmer with this action. If your butt muscle does not become firmer, bend deeper at your knee and trunk until it does. Now step your left foot forward and repeat with your left leg. Continue for 10–20 steps, gradually straightening your trunk and forward leg until you reach an upright position, with your knee almost straight. You will likely notice that your butt muscles turn off at some point as you straighten up. Continue practicing until, with your trunk in a fully upright position, you feel natural gluteal activation when your forward foot strikes the ground.

Once in a tall, upright position, gradually return to a "normal"-looking walk but with your gluteal muscles activating naturally (not consciously) with each foot strike.

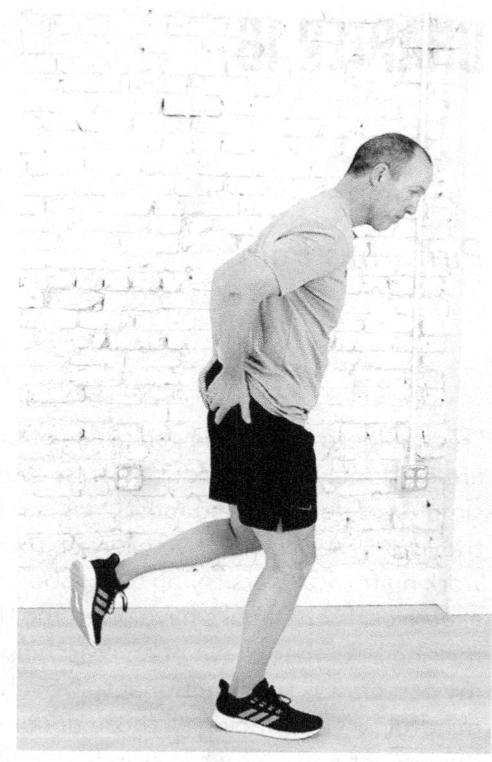

Mimicking ice-skating is a good way to activate your gluteal muscles to prepare for walking.

Gluteal Walking: Tiptoe Walking

Walk on your tiptoes for about 20 steps with your hands on your butt muscles. Feel that your butt muscles contract at each foot strike. This is not a conscious contraction but is instead one that occurs naturally. Then, slowly lower your heels back down and feel that your butt muscles continue to contract naturally as you take steps. Repeat throughout the day until, without needing to tiptoe walk first, you can walk with your gluteal muscles turning on naturally at each foot strike.

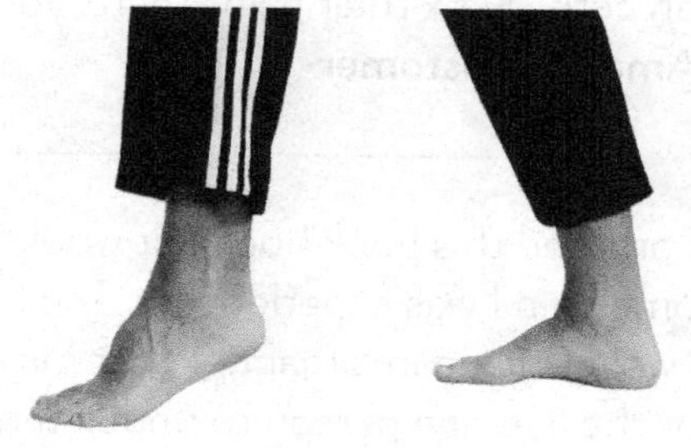

Tiptoe walking is a good way to activate your gluteal muscles to prepare for walking.

CHAPTER 16

Piriformis Pain

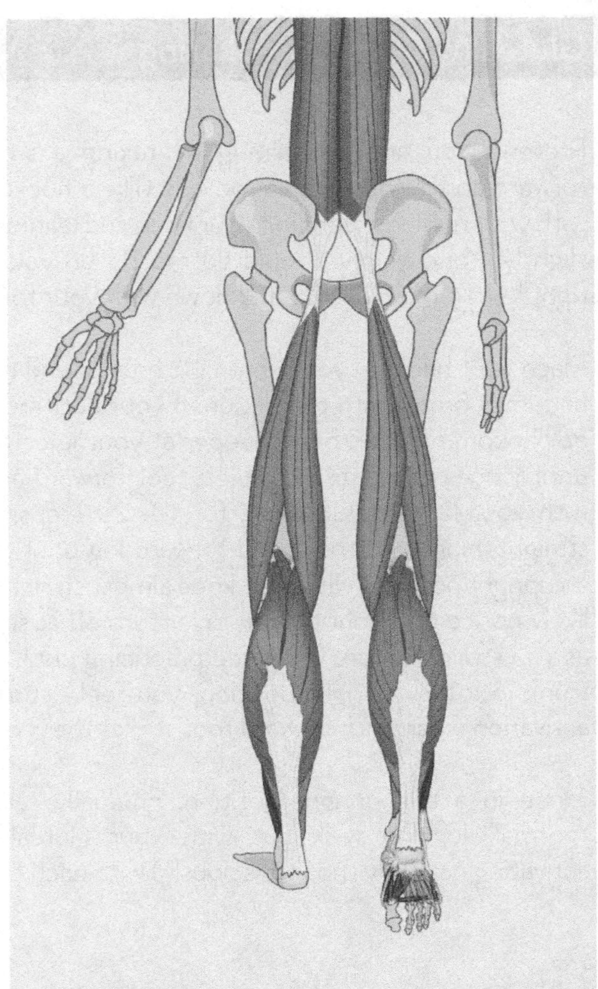

"Rick Olderman's *Fixing You* series of books are extremely good. Informative, practical, simple yet detailed, and most importantly, they work! As a corrective exercise therapist working for 25 years trying to fix bodies with exercises, Rick's books have given me the missing links that I have been searching for in my career. It is the functional approach, the mindfulness in noticing all those unconscious movement patterns while standing, walking, sitting, etc., and the positive approach to taking responsibility for one's own pain-free health and well-being. For many years, those in chronic pain are advised to accept their pain and to 'manage' their pain. Now, with awareness and targeted exercises, many people can actually fix their pain. Thank you, Rick!"
-Amazon Customer

"I ordered this book hoping it would help with some pain I was experiencing. The book itself is well-written in a manner that makes it easy for the average person to understand. Many other books I have found on the topic seem to overcomplicate things and use a bunch of medical jargon. The author does a good job explaining everything." **-Amazon Customer**

Pay special attention to asymmetries in strength, control, and range of motion. Your goals should include moving toward symmetry between the two legs.

Thigh Stretch

On a stable surface, such as a firm table or countertop, lie on your back with both knees drawn to your chest. Place a pillow under your head for additional comfort. Hold both knees with both hands to set your back and relax your legs.

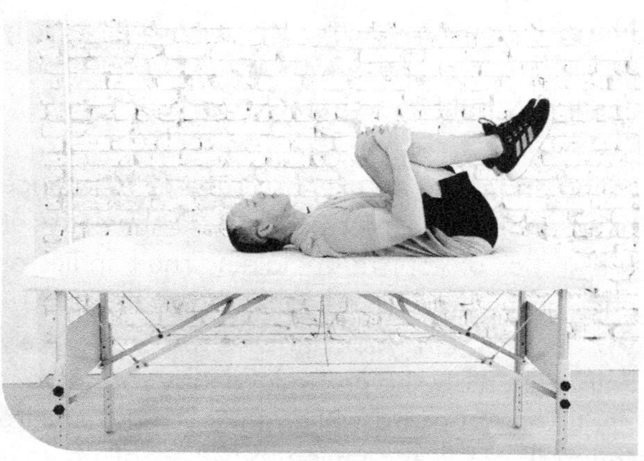

Hug both knees to your chest to set your back and pelvis.

Now, adjust your hands so they are both holding only your left knee. Slowly lower your right foot off the edge of the surface, keeping your right knee bent 90 degrees. Pull your left knee even closer to your chest to prevent your pelvis from rolling forward and your back from arching, as you lower your right leg down.

You should feel a stretch in your right upper thigh. Feel your leg gradually lower further as your muscles lengthen, but do not force your right leg down. If you have knee pain, move your right leg out so that your right knee is outside of your right hip. Over time, as your muscles lengthen, gradually move your leg back to the midline. Ideally, your right thigh should be able to rest on the surface, with your knee bent 90 degrees and positioned in line with your hip and shoulder. Hold for 7–10 breaths.

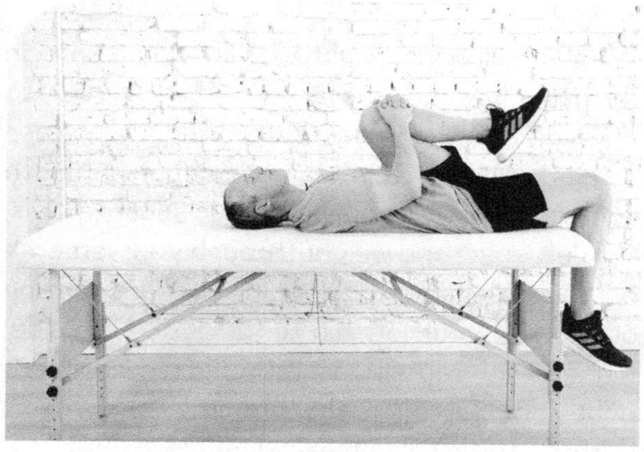

Hold your opposite knee close to your chest to protect your back and pelvis.

Bring your right leg back up to your chest and hug both knees to reset your back and pelvis. Repeat on the left side. Perform twice per side. Repeat 2–3 times per day.

Standing Hip Strengthening

Note: If you have difficulty balancing, initially perform this exercise without an exercise tube and lightly hold on to a stable surface.

Stand and place an exercise tube or resistance band under both feet, where your heels meet the arches of your feet. Holding the handles or ends of the band, bend your elbows about 80–90 degrees. Lift your right foot approximately half an inch off the ground. Slightly rotate your right knee outward while maintaining a square (neutral) pelvis and facing forward. Soften your left knee and make sure you are bearing weight through the arch or heel—not the toes—of your left foot.

While keeping your right foot lifted half an inch from the ground, move your right leg out to the side and then back in (moving about 6–8 inches). Make sure the movement is smooth and slow while maintaining your square pelvis, soft left knee, and weight through your left arch or heel. Maintain a tall spine without leaning or allowing your left hip to jut out to the side. Perform 15 repetitions without allowing your right foot to touch the ground. Switch legs. Perform three sets on each leg.

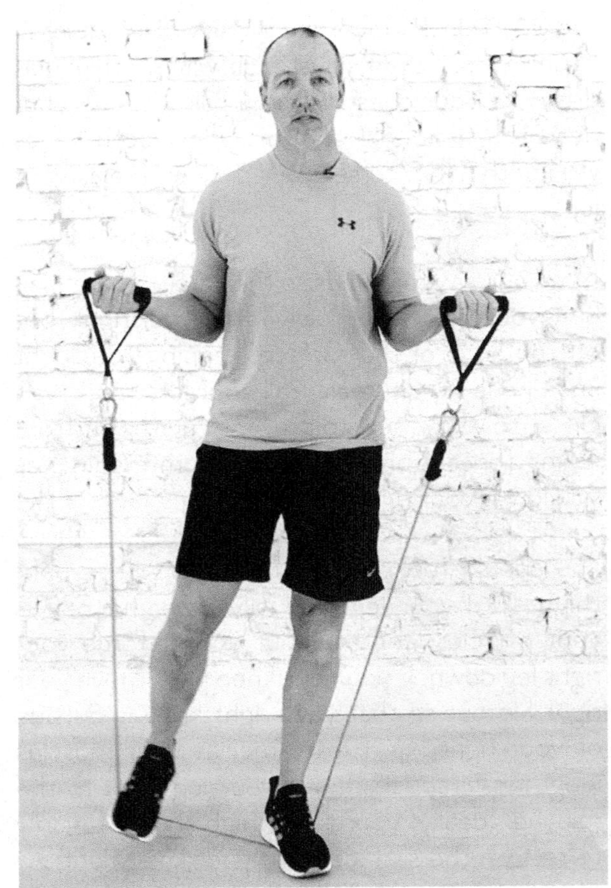

Maintain a soft stance knee and symmetrical upright posture during this exercise.

Butt Pumps

Assume a position on your elbows and knees with your lower spine flat, not sagging down toward the ground. Hold your lower spine in place by drawing in your belly button. Use your gluteals (butt muscles) to raise one leg in the air, with your knee bent 90 degrees. Stop at the point at which you feel the maximal contraction of your butt muscles. Do not overuse your low back or hamstring muscles to lift your leg.

Perform a small pump of your leg up and down (about 1–2 inches) while maintaining the gluteal contraction. Do not lower your leg so far that you feel your gluteal muscles turn off; they should remain activated throughout the exercise. Perform 10–30 repetitions, until your gluteals fatigue. Be sure not to recruit your back or hamstring muscles when performing this exercise.

If you don't feel your butt muscles contracting, rotate your knee out slightly until you do, and then perform the pump. Switch sides. Perform two sets per session. Perform 2–3 times per day.

• • •

Videos are available for all exercises and habit changes presented in this book. Go to the website top3fix.com and enter your email and the code TOP3FIX to access them.

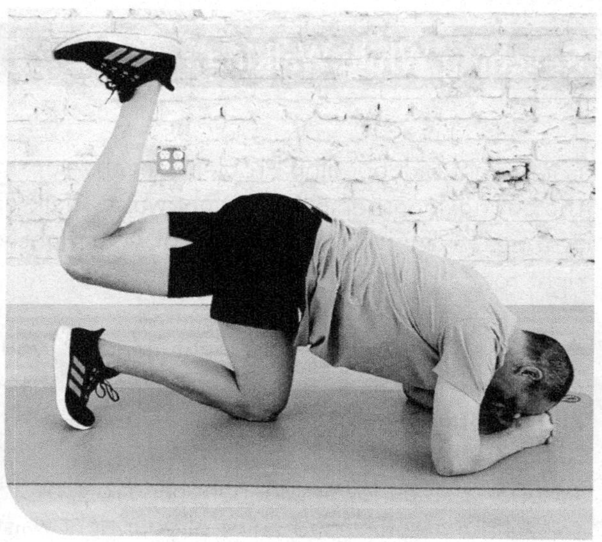

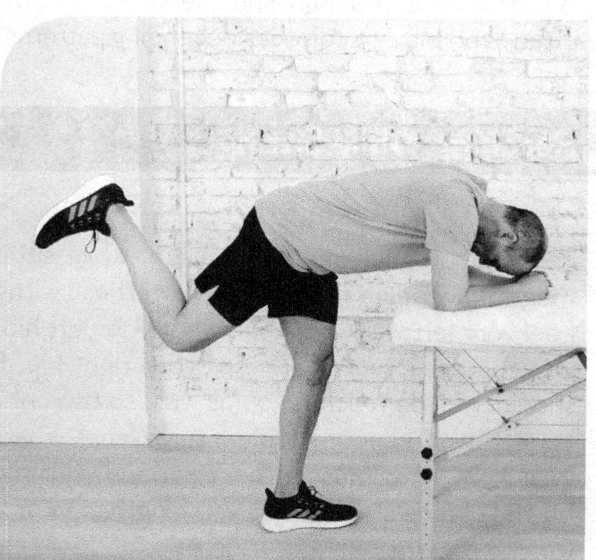

Gluteal strengthening is often the key to most lower body or back pain problems.

Fix Pain-Causing Habits

These exercises are designed to help fix dysfunctions in walking that lead to asymmetries and unilateral pain.

Reaching While Walking

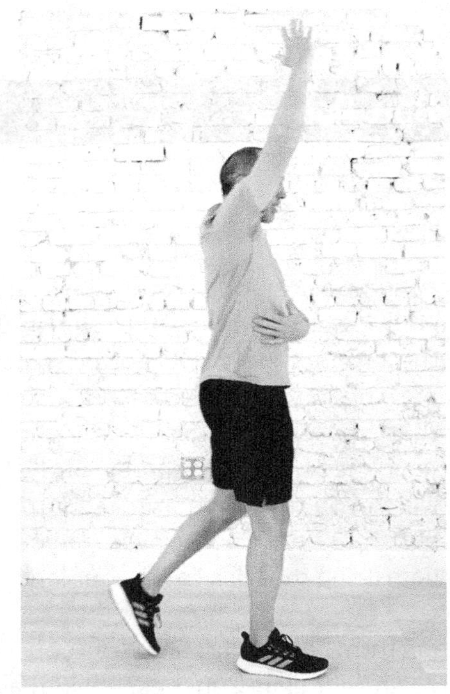

Learn to maintain a lengthened right waist while walking.

For a Right Sidebending Problem, reach your right arm up to the ceiling, lengthening your right waist. Walk with your right arm up, feeling the lengthening of your right waist at each right foot strike.

After 3–5 steps, rest your right hand on your head while continuing to walk, maintaining the length of your right waist and the engagement of your right gluteals.

After 3–5 steps, lower your right hand to your side, continuing to feel the natural lengthening of your right waist as you walk. Avoid hiking up your right shoulder to assist with this. Repeat as often as possible to correct sidebending patterns while walking.

Reaching While Sitting

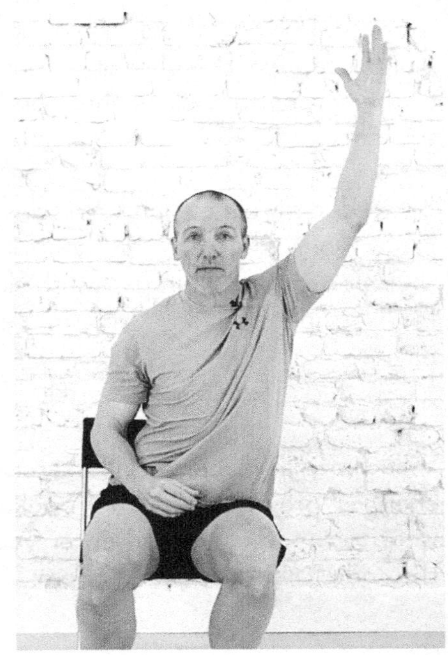

Learn to maintain a lengthened right waist while sitting.

For a Right Sidebending Problem, while sitting, shift your weight to your left hip and reach overhead with your left arm. Feel your left waist lengthen while your left hip pushes down into the chair seat relative to your right hip. Feel your left shoulder blade reaching up as well, so the entire left side of your trunk and your shoulder have lengthened. Notice that your right waist muscles contract and your right hip comes off the chair a little to help you lengthen your left side. Hold for two breaths.

Perform on the right side. Repeat on both sides, finishing with the right side to train your body to lengthen on the right side while sitting. Repeat frequently when sitting.

Gluteal Walking: Ice-Skating

Pretend you are ice-skating by taking a small lunge forward and slightly out to the side (like a hockey player) with your right leg, bending your knee and leaning forward slightly. Your weight should be mostly on your forward right leg. Pump twice up and down with your forward leg.

Place your hand on your right butt muscle and feel that it becomes firmer with this action. If your butt muscle does not become firmer, bend deeper at your knee and trunk until it does. Now step your left foot forward and repeat with your left leg. Continue for 10–20 steps, gradually straightening your trunk and forward leg until you reach an upright position, with your knee almost straight. You will likely notice that your butt muscles turn off at some point, as you straighten up. Continue practicing until, with your trunk in a fully upright position, you feel natural gluteal activation when your forward foot strikes the ground.

Once you are in a tall, upright position, gradually return to a "normal"-looking walk but with your gluteal muscles activating naturally (not consciously) with each foot strike.

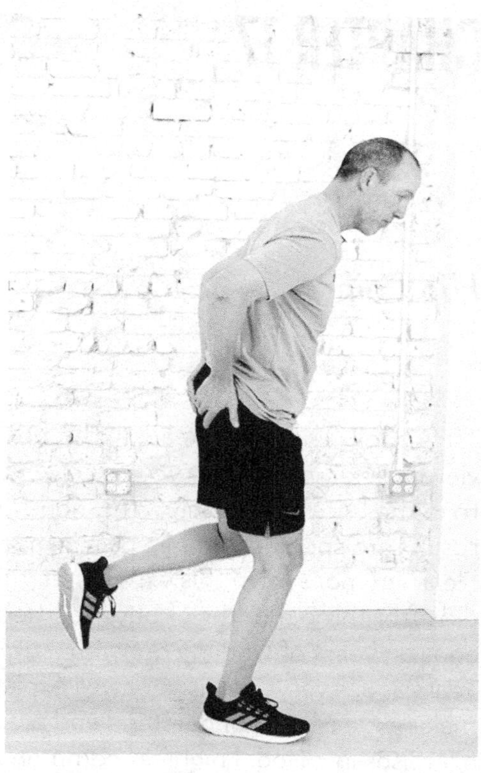

Mimicking ice-skating is a good way to activate your gluteal muscles to prepare for walking.

Gluteal Walking: Tiptoe Walking

Walk on your tiptoes for about 20 steps with your hands on your butt muscles. Feel that your butt muscles contract at each foot strike. This is not a conscious contraction but is instead one that occurs naturally. Then, slowly lower your heels back down and feel that your butt muscles continue to contract naturally as you take steps. Repeat throughout the day until, without needing to tiptoe walk first, you can walk with your gluteal muscles turning on naturally at each foot strike.

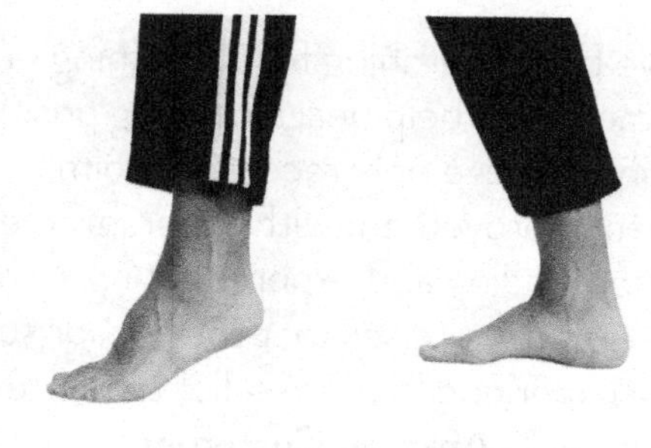

Tiptoe walking is a good way to activate your gluteal muscles to prepare for walking.

CHAPTER 17

Hip Pain

"This book is right on. Reading this book and viewing the videos (that you are given the link to in the book) takes only a few hours and the results are spectacular. Hip pain is much better. I learned more from this experience than I did after three months of physical therapy and ten years of working out with a trainer years ago. Everything is very well explained, making it easier to understand and practice the exercises involved. I highly recommend this book to anyone motivated to fix their pain. For anyone undergoing physical therapy, this book is a great adjuvant, explaining how and why exercises work, which encourages compliance and leads to real success." **-Amazon Customer**

"I've been searching for something or someone to help heal a nagging positional hip pain and have only received minimal short-term improvement with other interventions. After reading and experimenting with the tests and exercises that the author suggests, I've experienced more relief than I've had in months." **-Amazon Customer**

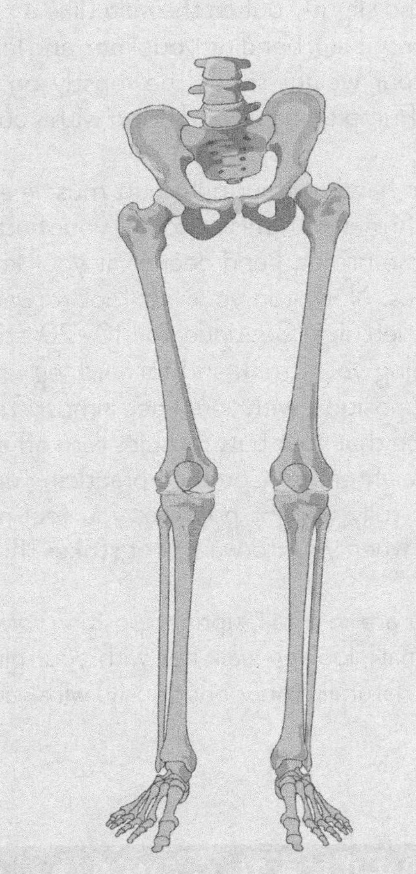

Pay special attention to asymmetries in strength, control, and range of motion. Your goals should include moving toward symmetry between your two legs.

Thigh Stretch

On a stable surface, such as a firm table or countertop, lie on your back with both knees drawn to your chest. Place a pillow under your head for additional comfort. Hold both knees with both hands to set your back and relax your legs.

Now, adjust your hands so they are both holding only your left knee. Slowly lower your right foot off the edge of the surface, keeping your right knee bent 90 degrees. Pull your left knee even closer to your chest to prevent your pelvis from rolling forward and your back from arching, as you lower your right leg down.

You should feel a stretch in your right upper thigh. Feel your leg gradually lower further as your muscles lengthen, but do not force your right leg down. If you have knee pain, move your right leg out so that your right knee is outside of your right hip. Over time, as your muscles lengthen, gradually move your leg back to midline. Ideally, your right thigh should be able to rest on the surface, with your knee bent 90 degrees and positioned in line with your hip and shoulder. Hold for 7–10 breaths.

Bring your right leg back up to your chest and hug both knees to reset your back and pelvis. Repeat on the left side. Perform twice per side. Repeat 2–3 times per day.

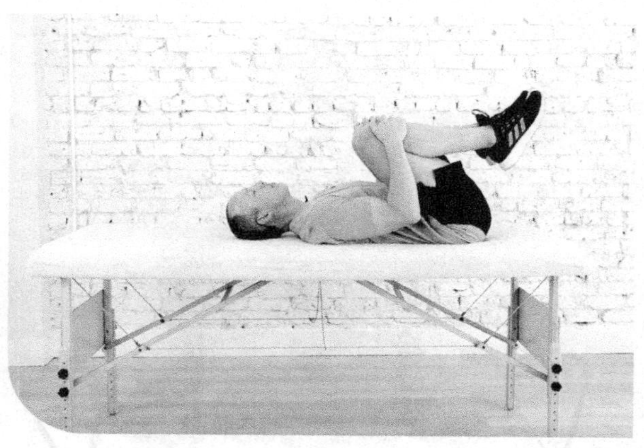

Hug both knees to your chest to set your back and pelvis.

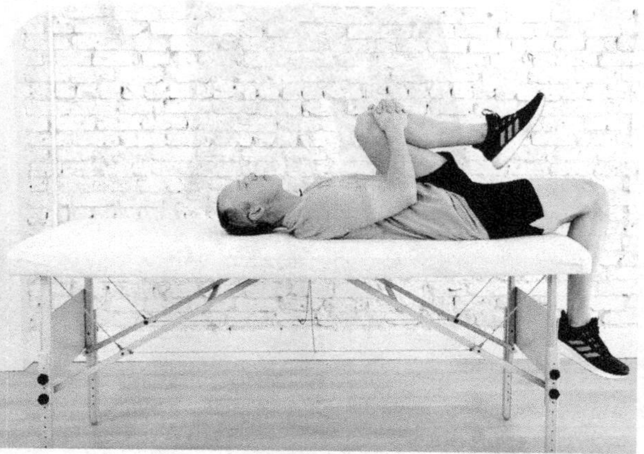

Hold your opposite knee close to your chest to protect your back and pelvis.

Standing Hip Strengthening

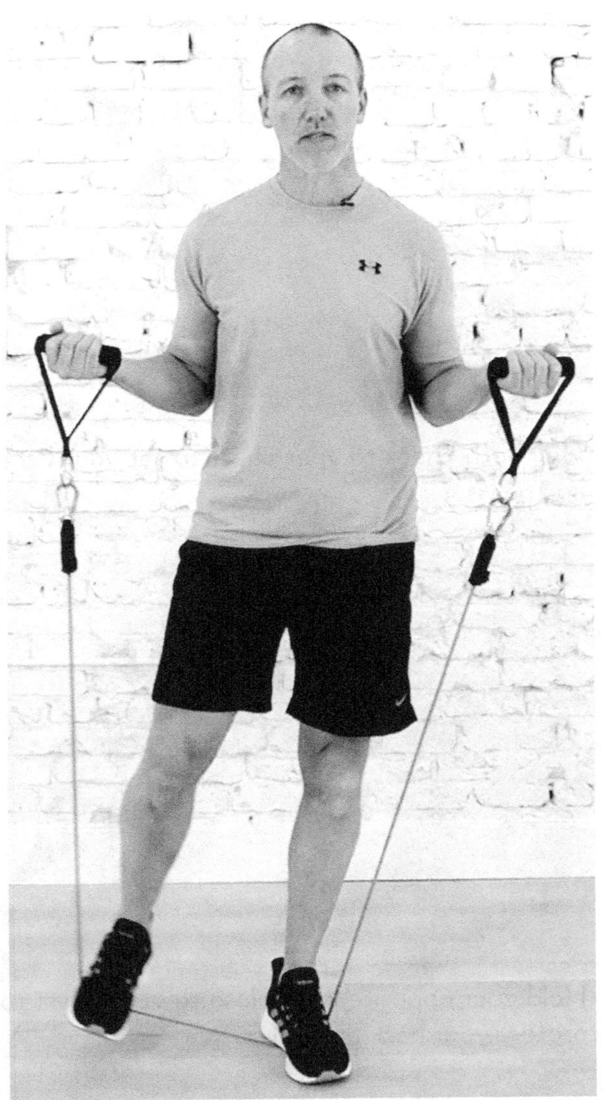

Maintain a soft stance knee and symmetrical upright posture during this exercise.

Note: If you have difficulty balancing, initially perform this exercise without an exercise tube and lightly hold on to a stable surface.

Stand and place an exercise tube or resistance band under both feet, where your heels meet the arches of your feet. Holding the handles or ends of the band, bend your elbows about 80–90 degrees. Lift your right foot approximately half an inch off the ground. Slightly rotate your right knee outward, while maintaining a square (neutral) pelvis and facing forward. Soften your left knee and make sure you are bearing weight through the arch or heel—not the toes—of your left foot.

While keeping your right foot lifted half an inch from the ground, move your right leg out to the side and then back in (moving about 6–8 inches). Make sure the movement is smooth and slow while maintaining your square pelvis, soft left knee, and weight through your left arch or heel. Maintain a tall spine without leaning or allowing your left hip to jut out to the side. Perform 15 repetitions without allowing your right foot to touch the ground. Switch legs. Perform three sets on each leg.

Butt Pumps

Assume a position on your elbows and knees with your lower spine flat, not sagging down toward the ground. Hold your lower spine in place by drawing in your belly button. Use your gluteals (butt muscles) to raise one leg in the air with your knee bent 90 degrees. Stop at the point at which you feel the maximal contraction of your butt muscles. Do not overuse your low back or hamstring muscles to lift your leg.

Perform a small pump of your leg up and down (about 1–2 inches) while maintaining the gluteal contraction. Do not lower your leg so far that you feel your gluteal muscles turn off; they should remain activated throughout the exercise. Perform 10–30 repetitions, until your gluteals fatigue. Be sure not to recruit your back or hamstring muscles when performing this exercise.

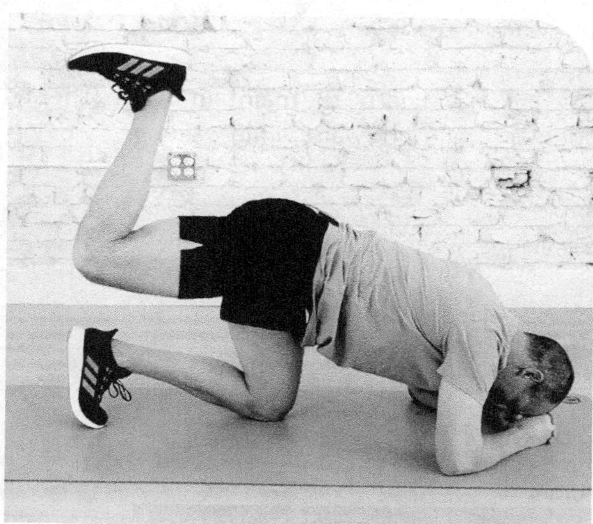

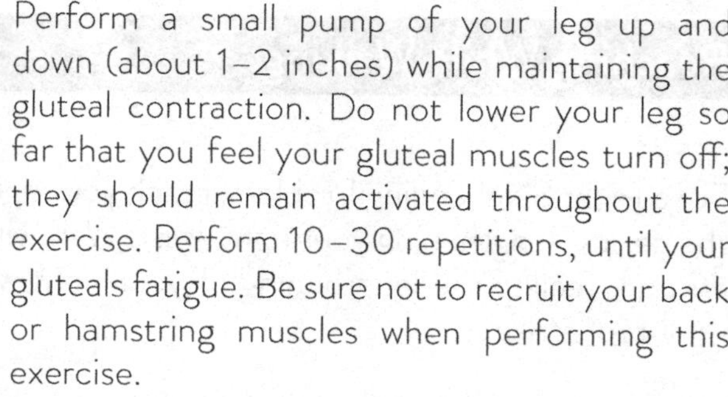

Gluteal strengthening is often the key to most lower body or back pain problems.

If you don't feel your butt muscles contracting, rotate your knee out slightly until you do, and then perform the pump. Switch sides. Perform two sets per session. Perform 2–3 times per day.

• • •

Videos are available for all exercises and habit changes presented in this book. Go to the website top3fix.com and enter your email and the code TOP3FIX to access them.

Fix Pain-Causing Habits

These exercises are designed to help fix dysfunctions in walking that lead to asymmetries and unilateral pain.

Reaching While Walking

For a Right Sidebending Problem, reach your right arm up to the ceiling, lengthening your right waist. Walk with your right arm up, feeling the lengthening of your right waist at each right foot strike.

After 3–5 steps, rest your right hand on your head while continuing to walk, maintaining the length of your right waist and the engagement of your right gluteals.

After 3–5 steps, lower your right hand to your side, continuing to feel the natural lengthening of your right waist as you walk. Avoid hiking up your right shoulder to assist with this. Repeat as often as possible to correct sidebending patterns while walking.

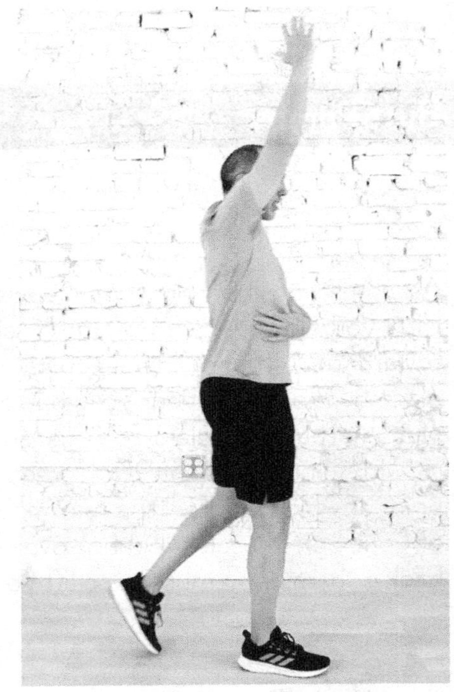

Learn to maintain a lengthened right waist while walking.

Reaching While Sitting

For a Right Sidebending Problem, while sitting, shift your weight to your left hip and reach overhead with your left arm. Feel your left waist lengthen while your left hip pushes down into the chair seat relative to your right hip. Feel your left shoulder blade reaching up as well, so the entire left side of your trunk and your shoulder have lengthened. Notice that your right waist muscles contract and your right hip comes off the chair a little to help you lengthen your left side. Hold for two breaths.

Perform on the right side. Repeat on both sides, finishing with the right side to train your body to lengthen on the right side while sitting. Repeat frequently when sitting.

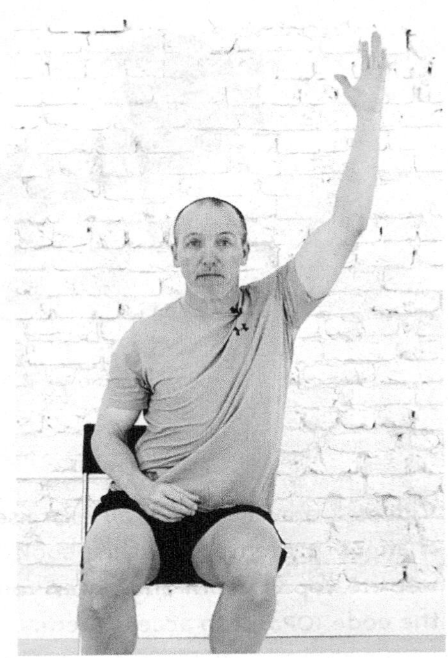

Learn to maintain a lengthened right waist while sitting.

Gluteal Walking: Ice-Skating

Pretend you are ice-skating by taking a small lunge forward and slightly out to the side (like a hockey player) with your right leg, bending your knee and leaning forward slightly. Your weight should be mostly on your forward right leg. Pump twice up and down with your forward leg.

Place your hand on your right butt muscle and feel that it becomes firmer with this action. If your butt muscle does not become firmer, bend deeper at your knee and trunk until it does. Now step your left foot forward and repeat with your left leg. Continue for 10–20 steps, gradually straightening your trunk and forward leg until you reach an upright position, with your knee almost straight. You will likely notice that your butt muscles turn off at some point, as you straighten up. Continue practicing until, with your trunk in a fully upright position, you feel natural gluteal activation when your forward foot strikes the ground.

Once you are in a tall, upright position, gradually return to a "normal"-looking walk but with your gluteal muscles activating naturally (not consciously) with each foot strike.

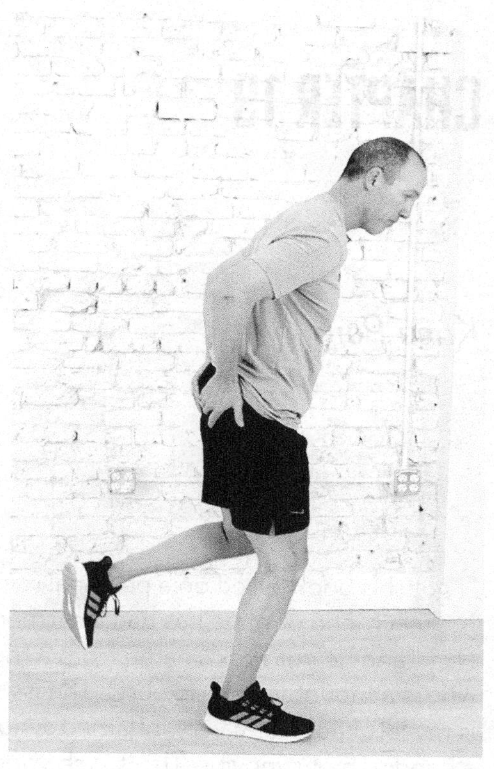

Mimicking ice-skating is a good way to activate your gluteal muscles to prepare for walking.

Gluteal Walking: Tiptoe Walking

Walk on your tiptoes for about 20 steps with your hands on your butt muscles. Feel that your butt muscles contract at each foot strike. This is not a conscious contraction but is instead one that occurs naturally. Then, slowly lower your heels back down and feel that your butt muscles continue to contract naturally as you take steps. Repeat throughout the day until, without needing to tiptoe walk first, you can walk with your gluteal muscles turning on naturally at each foot strike.

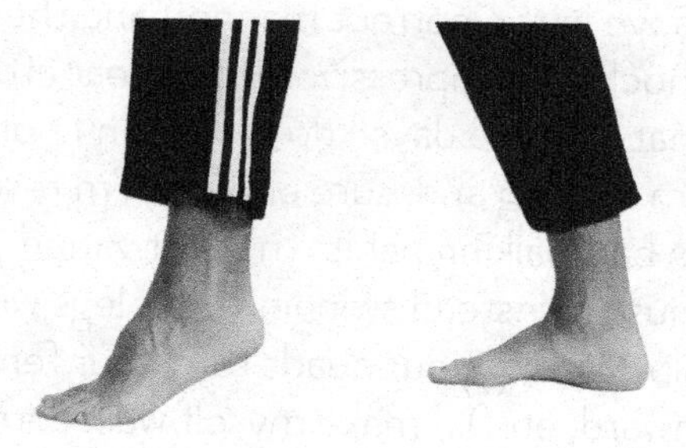

Tiptoe walking is a good way to activate your gluteal muscles to prepare for walking.

CHAPTER 18

Knee Pain

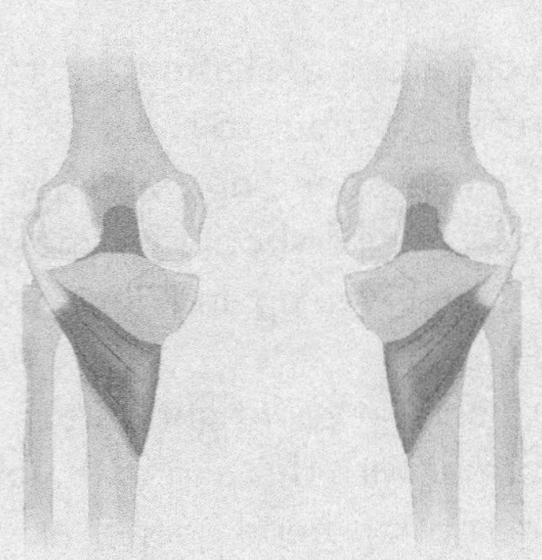

"I got this book based on a personal review of Rick. A friend of mine has had treatment from Rick (and he got Rick's name from a friend of his who is a mountain bike expert). The issue I have is my left knee has a very inflamed synovium, a condition of synovitis. The 'teach yourself how to walk' part of this book was great. I didn't think that how I was walking was contributing to this condition, however it was completely contributing to it. I started doing the exercises in the book, which feel awkward because they are using muscles you rarely use, and making myself move in the correct manner, and the results are shockingly impressive. I feel great after doing that. On the days I do have pain I notice how I'm moving and, sure enough, I'm resorting back to bad walking habits (not activating your butt muscle, instead swinging your legs with your hips, letting your quads turn your femur slightly inward, etc.). I make myself walk correctly and my pain is gone. Great book, great physical therapist/teacher." **-Amazon Customer**

"I started doing the exercises recommended here a week ago. They have made an appreciable difference in my knee pain, and it should continue to improve. Also, some of the exercises can be adapted so you can do them standing up, and I take a few minutes to do them while engaged in other tasks like washing the dishes or waiting for the train. I'm now really confident I can go hiking in Europe again next year. Thank you, Rick!" **-Amazon Customer**

Pay special attention to asymmetries in strength, control, and range of motion. Your goals should include moving toward symmetry between the two legs.

Thigh Stretch

On a stable surface, such as a firm table or countertop, lie on your back with both knees drawn to your chest. Place a pillow under your head for additional comfort. Hold both knees with both hands to set your back and relax your legs.

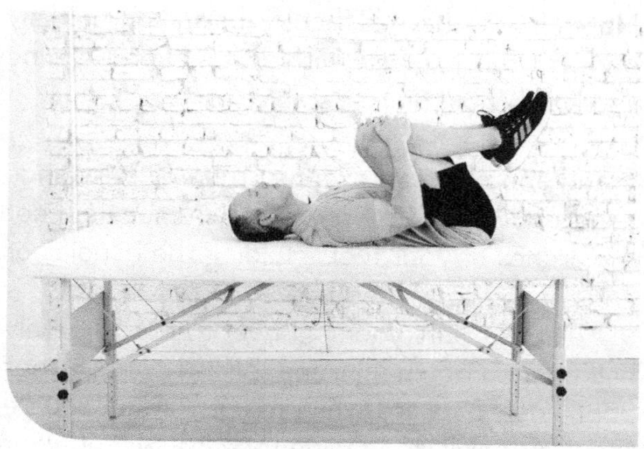

Hug both knees to your chest to set your back and pelvis.

Now, adjust your hands so they are both holding only your left knee. Slowly lower your right foot off the edge of the surface, keeping your right knee bent 90 degrees. Pull your left knee even closer to your chest, to prevent your pelvis from rolling forward and your back from arching as you lower your right leg down.

You should feel a stretch in your right upper thigh. Feel your leg gradually lower further as your muscles lengthen, but do not force your right leg down. If you have knee pain, move your right leg out so that your right knee is outside of your right hip. Over time, as your muscles lengthen, gradually move your leg back to the midline. Ideally, your right thigh should be able to rest on the surface with your knee bent 90 degrees and positioned in line with your hip and shoulder. Hold for 7–10 breaths.

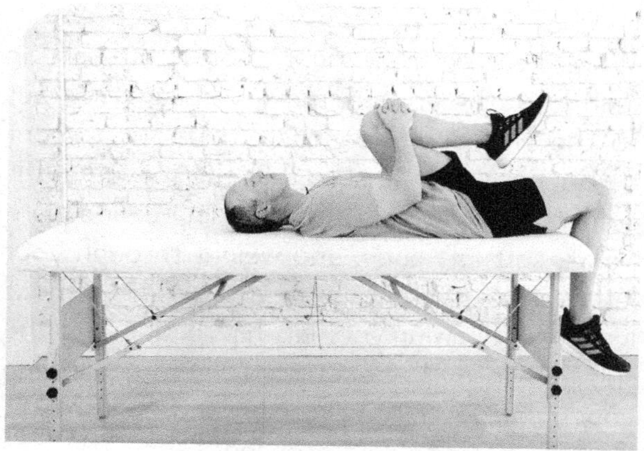

Hold your opposite knee close to your chest to protect your back and pelvis.

Bring your right leg back up to your chest and hug both knees, to reset your back and pelvis. Repeat on the left side. Perform twice per side. Repeat 2–3 times per day.

Standing Hip Strengthening

Note: If you have difficulty balancing, initially perform this exercise without an exercise tube and lightly hold on to a stable surface.

Stand and place an exercise tube or resistance band under both feet, where your heels meet the arches of your feet. Holding the handles or ends of the band, bend your elbows about 80–90 degrees. Lift your right foot approximately half an inch off the ground. Slightly rotate your right knee outward while maintaining a square (neutral) pelvis and facing forward. Soften your left knee and make sure you are bearing weight through the arch or heel—not the toes—of your left foot.

While keeping your right foot lifted half an inch from the ground, move your right leg out to the side and then back in (moving about 6–8 inches). Make sure that the movement is smooth and slow while maintaining your square pelvis, soft left knee, and weight through your left arch or heel. Maintain a tall spine without leaning or allowing your left hip to jut out to the side. Perform 15 repetitions without allowing your right foot to touch the ground. Switch legs. Perform three sets on each leg.

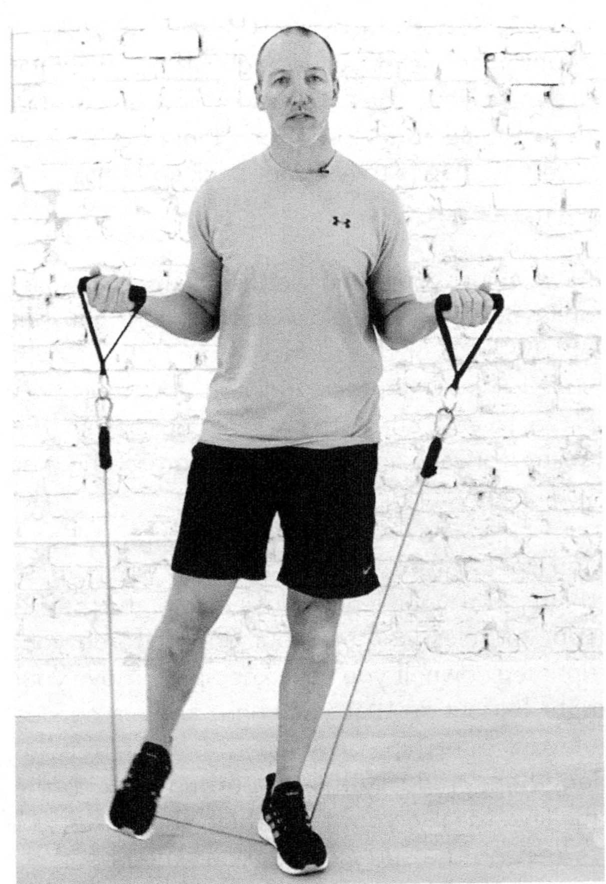

Maintain a soft stance knee and symmetrical upright posture during this exercise.

Butt Pumps

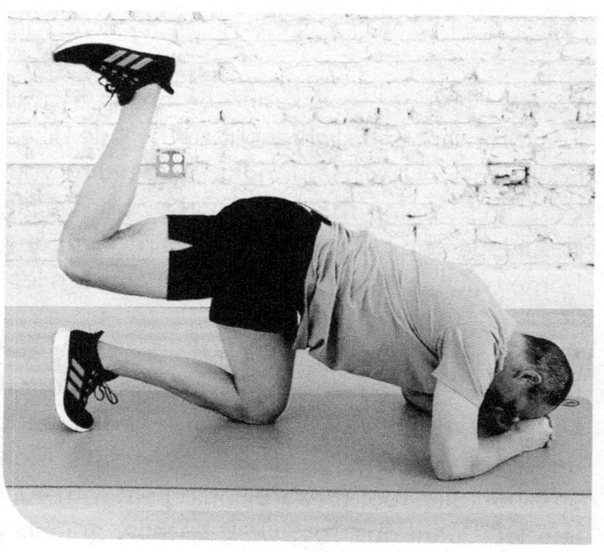

Assume a position on your elbows and knees with your lower spine flat, not sagging down toward the ground. Hold your lower spine in place by drawing in your belly button. Use your gluteals (butt muscles) to raise one leg in the air with your knee bent 90 degrees. Stop at the point at which you feel the maximal contraction of your butt muscles. Do not overuse your low back or hamstring muscles to lift your leg.

Perform a small pump of your leg up and down (about 1–2 inches) while maintaining the gluteal contraction. Do not lower your leg so far that you feel your gluteal muscles turn off. They should remain activated throughout the exercise. Perform 10–30 repetitions, until your gluteals fatigue. Be sure not to recruit your back or hamstring muscles when performing this exercise.

If you don't feel your butt muscles contracting, rotate your knee out slightly until you do, and then perform the pump. Switch sides. Perform two sets per session. Perform 2–3 times per day.

• • •

Videos are available for all exercises and habit changes presented in this book. Go to the website top3fix.com and enter your email and the code TOP3FIX to access them.

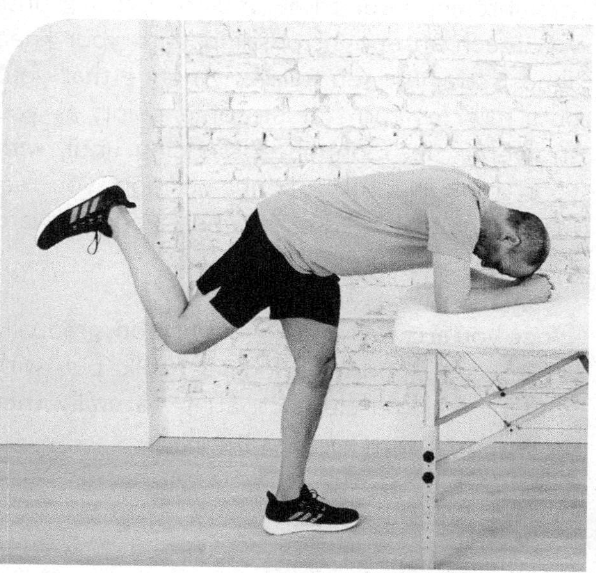

Gluteal strengthening is often the key to most lower body or back pain problems.

Fix Pain-Causing Habits

Gluteal Walking: Ice-Skating

Pretend you are ice-skating by taking a small lunge forward and slightly out to the side (like a hockey player) with your right leg, bending your knee and leaning forward slightly. Your weight should be mostly on your forward right leg. Pump twice up and down with your forward leg.

Place your hand on your right butt muscle and feel that it becomes firmer with this action. If your butt muscle does not become firmer, bend deeper at your knee and trunk until it does. Now step your left foot forward and repeat with your left leg. Continue for 10–20 steps, gradually straightening your trunk and forward leg until you reach an upright position, with your knee almost straight. You will likely notice that your butt muscles turn off at some point, as you straighten up. Continue practicing until, with your trunk in a fully upright position, you feel natural gluteal activation when your forward foot strikes the ground.

Once you are in a tall, upright position, gradually return to a "normal"-looking walk but with your gluteal muscles activating naturally (not consciously) with each foot strike.

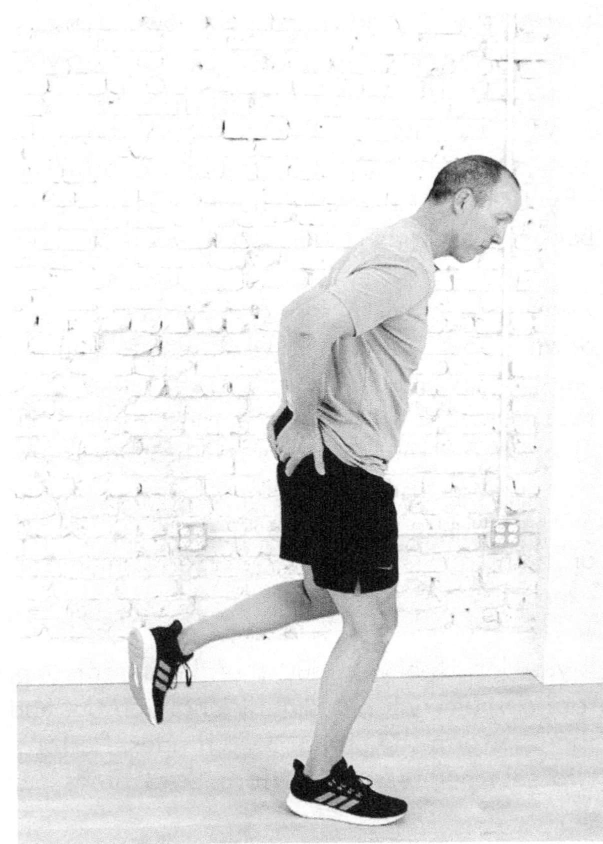

Mimicking ice-skating is a good way to activate your gluteal muscles to prepare for walking.

Gluteal Walking: Tiptoe Walking

Walk on your tiptoes for about 20 steps with your hands on your butt muscles. Feel that your butt muscles contract at each foot strike. This is not a conscious contraction but is instead one that occurs naturally. Then, slowly lower your heels back down and feel that your butt muscles continue to contract naturally as you take steps. Repeat throughout the day until, without needing to tiptoe walk first, you can walk with your gluteal muscles turning on naturally at each foot strike.

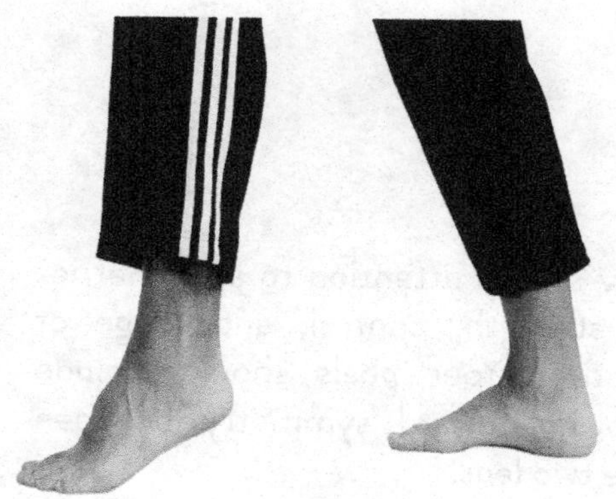

Tiptoe walking is a good way to activate your gluteal muscles to prepare for walking.

Dorsal Night Splint

The calf/soleus muscle complex in the lower leg crosses the knee joint and, when tight, contributes to knee pain. This tightness typically occurs because of sleeping habits that point the toes down, placing the ankle in a position of plantarflexion. This shortens the calf/soleus complex for 6–8 hours, wiping away any lengthening that occurs during the day.

Wear a dorsal splint at night to hold the ankle in a neutral position while sleeping, maintaining the length of the calf/soleus complex. This will reduce the forces acting on the knee joint.

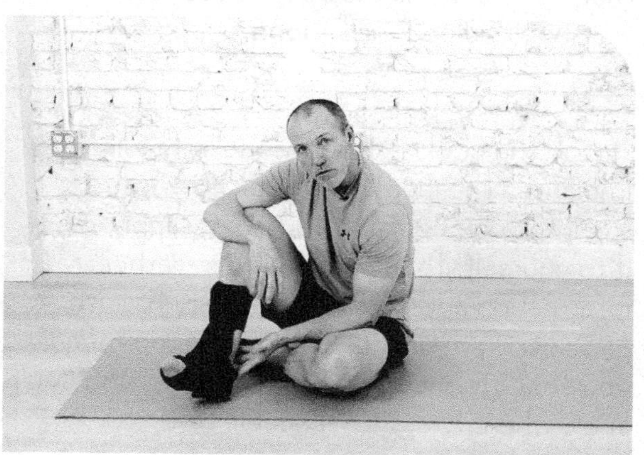

A dorsal night splint reduces the shortening of the calf/soleus complex that occurs while sleeping.

CHAPTER 19

Plantar Fasciitis

"This book gives you the information you need to diagnose your foot and ankle pain. I found it more helpful than physical therapy. It also gives you helpful exercises and a method of walking that lessens the stress on the foot during walking. It helped me." **-John B**

"I read the book in one day and immediately implanted the ideas. This book gives you the info you need, and you simply apply it to yourself. The book really just gathers information and puts you on the right path. I also liked the online videos. I'd recommend you check it out if you have foot pain and don't know where to start." **-Daniele S**

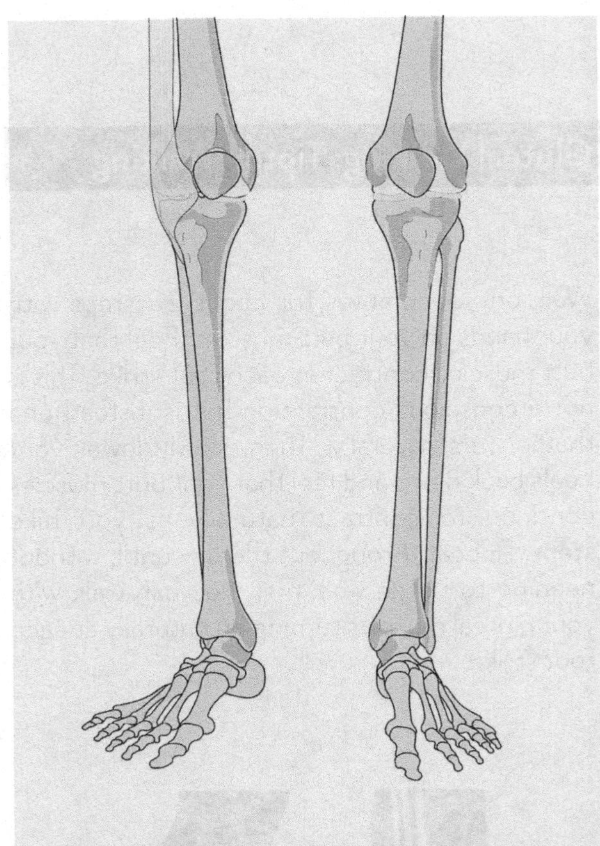

Pay special attention to asymmetries in strength, control, and range of motion. Your goals should include moving toward symmetry between the two legs.

Thigh Stretch

On a stable surface, such as a firm table or countertop, lie on your back with both knees drawn to your chest. Place a pillow under your head for additional comfort. Hold both knees with both hands to set your back and relax your legs.

Now, adjust your hands so they are both holding only your left knee. Slowly lower your right foot off the edge of the surface, keeping your right knee bent 90 degrees. Pull your left knee even closer to your chest, to prevent your pelvis from rolling forward and your back from arching as you lower your right leg down.

You should feel a stretch in your right upper thigh. Feel your leg gradually lower further as your muscles lengthen, but do not force your right leg down. If you have knee pain, move your right leg out so that your right knee is outside of your right hip. Over time, as your muscles lengthen, gradually move your leg back to midline. Ideally, your right thigh should be able to rest on the surface with your knee bent 90 degrees and positioned in line with your hip and shoulder. Hold for 7–10 breaths.

Bring your right leg back up to your chest and hug both knees to reset your back and pelvis. Repeat on the left side. Perform twice per side. Repeat 2–3 times per day.

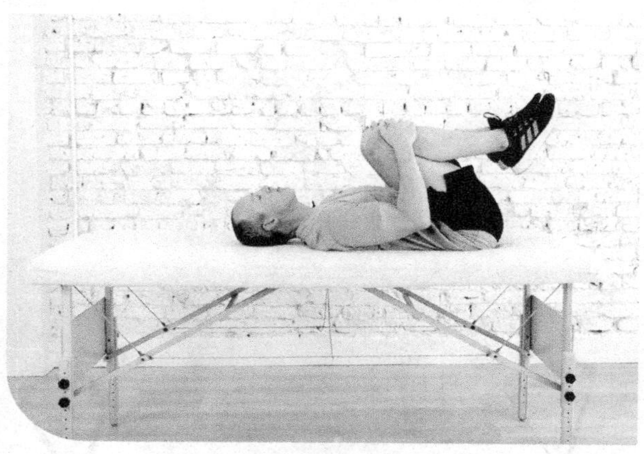

Hug both knees to your chest to set your back and pelvis.

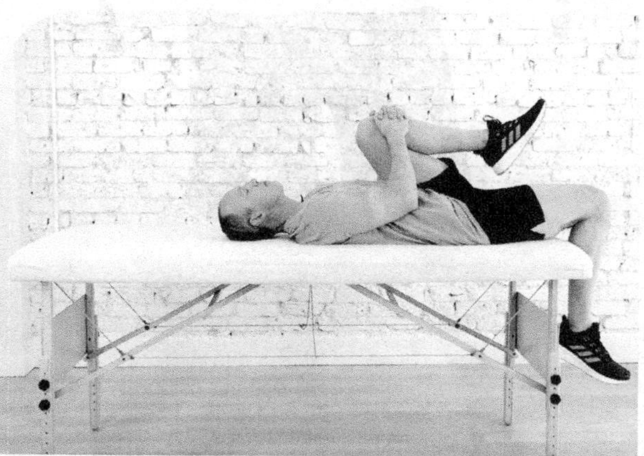

Hold your opposite knee close to your chest to protect your back and pelvis.

Standing Hip Strengthening

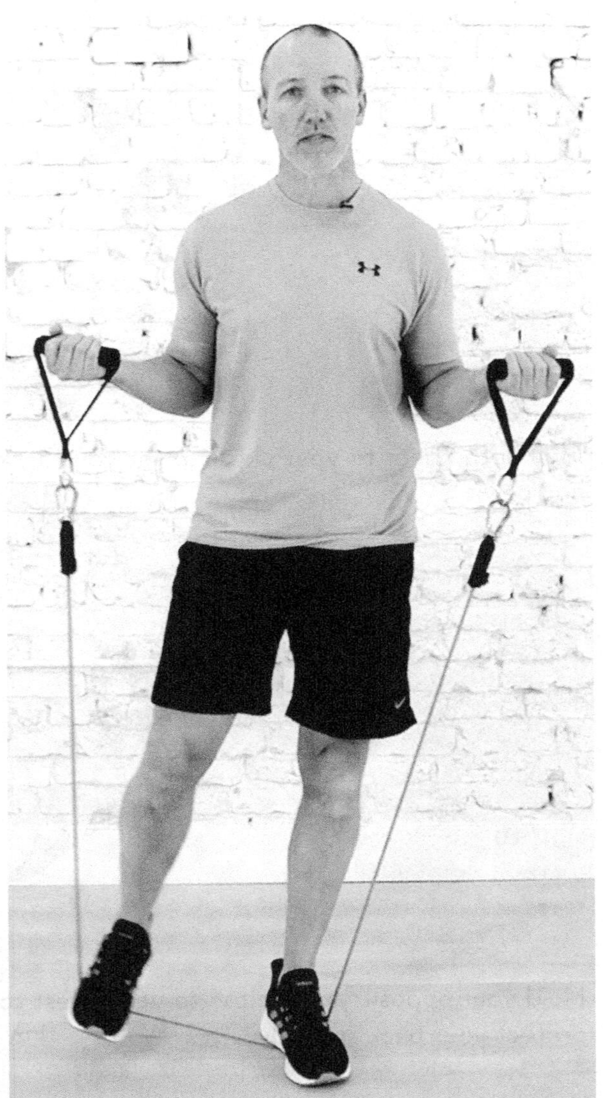

Maintain a soft stance knee and symmetrical upright posture during this exercise.

Note: If you have difficulty balancing, initially perform this exercise without an exercise tube and lightly hold on to a stable surface.

Stand and place an exercise tube or resistance band under both feet where your heels meet the arches of your feet. Holding the handles or ends of the band, bend your elbows about 80–90 degrees. Lift your right foot approximately half an inch off the ground. Slightly rotate your right knee outward while maintaining a square (neutral) pelvis and facing forward. Soften your left knee and make sure you are bearing weight through the arch or heel—not the toes—of your left foot.

While keeping your right foot lifted half an inch from the ground, move your right leg out to the side and then back in (moving about 6–8 inches). Make sure the movement is smooth and slow while maintaining your square pelvis, soft left knee, and weight through your left arch or heel. Maintain a tall spine without leaning or allowing your left hip to jut out to the side. Perform 15 repetitions without allowing your right foot to touch the ground. Switch legs. Perform three sets on each leg.

Butt Pumps

Assume a position on your elbows and knees with your lower spine flat, not sagging down toward the ground. Hold your lower spine in place by drawing in your belly button. Use your gluteals (butt muscles) to raise one leg in the air, with your knee bent 90 degrees. Stop at the point at which you feel the maximal contraction of your butt muscles. Do not overuse your low back or hamstring muscles to lift your leg.

Perform a small pump of your leg up and down (about 1–2 inches) while maintaining the gluteal contraction. Do not lower your leg so far that you feel your gluteal muscles turn off. They should remain activated throughout the exercise. Perform 10–30 repetitions, until your gluteals fatigue. Be sure not to recruit your back or hamstring muscles when performing this exercise.

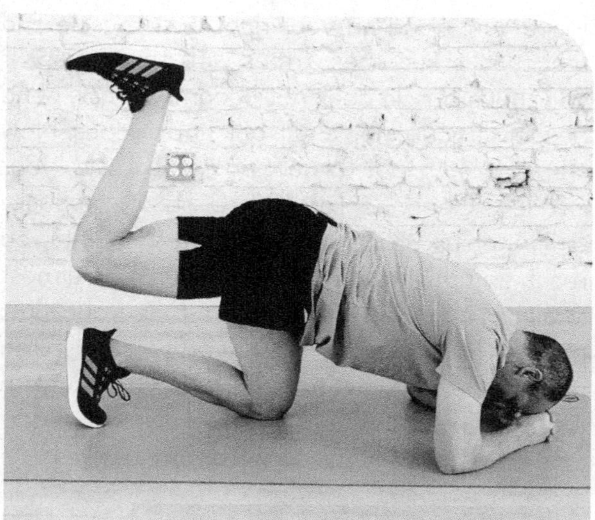

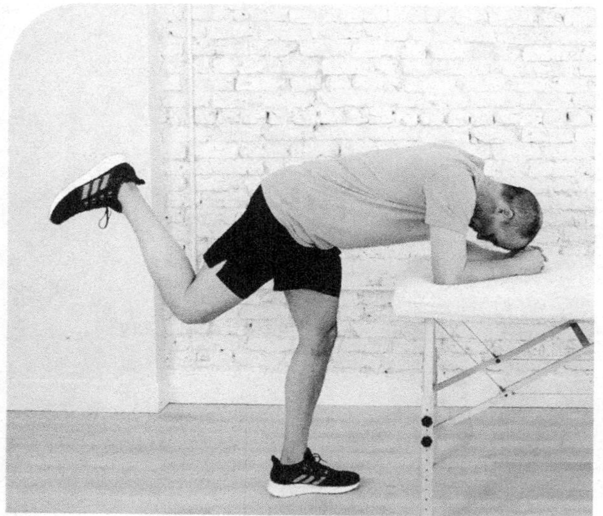

Gluteal strengthening is often the key to most lower body or back pain problems.

If you don't feel your butt muscles contracting, rotate your knee out slightly until you do, and then perform the pump. Switch sides. Perform two sets per session. Perform 2–3 times per day.

• • •

Videos are available for all exercises and habit changes presented in this book. Go to the website top3fix.com and enter your email and the code TOP3FIX to access them.

Fix Pain-Causing Habits

Gluteal Walking: Ice-Skating

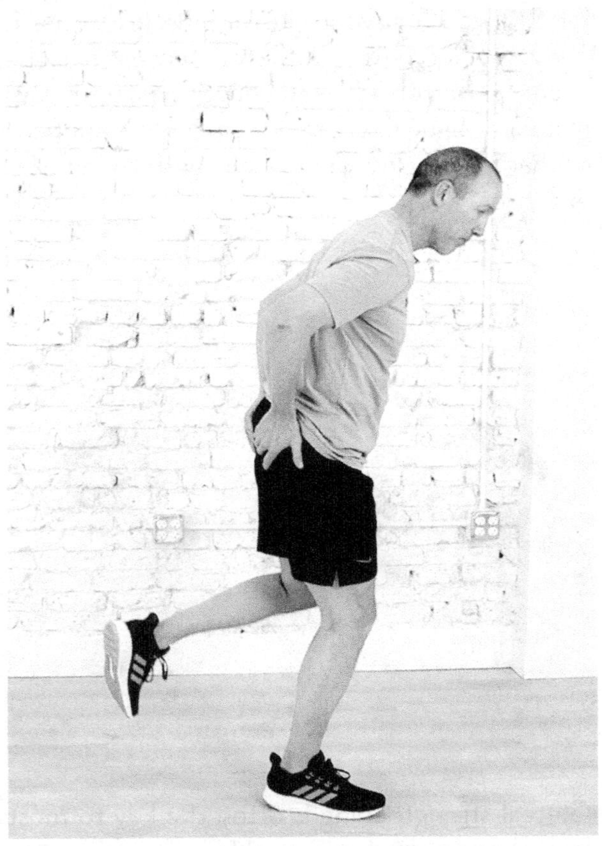

Mimicking ice-skating is a good way to activate your gluteal muscles to prepare for walking.

Pretend you are ice-skating by taking a small lunge forward and slightly out to the side (like a hockey player) with your right leg, bending your knee and leaning forward slightly. Your weight should be mostly on your forward right leg. Pump twice up and down with your forward leg.

Place your hand on your right butt muscle and feel that it becomes firmer with this action. If your butt muscle does not become firmer, bend deeper at your knee and trunk until it does. Now step your left foot forward and repeat with your left leg. Continue for 10–20 steps, gradually straightening your trunk and forward leg until you reach an upright position, with your knee almost straight. You will likely notice that your butt muscles turn off at some point, as you straighten up. Continue practicing until, with your trunk in a fully upright position, you feel natural gluteal activation when your forward foot strikes the ground.

Once you are in a tall, upright position, gradually return to a "normal"-looking walk but with your gluteal muscles activating naturally (not consciously) with each foot strike.

Gluteal Walking: Tiptoe Walking

Walk on your tiptoes for about 20 steps with your hands on your butt muscles. Feel that your butt muscles contract at each foot strike. This is not a conscious contraction but is instead one that occurs naturally. Then, slowly lower your heels back down and feel that your butt muscles continue to contract naturally as you take steps. Repeat throughout the day until, without needing to tiptoe walk first, you can walk with your gluteal muscles turning on naturally at each foot strike.

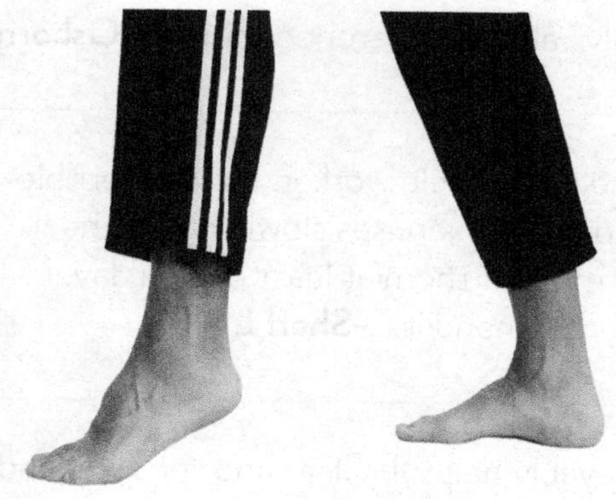

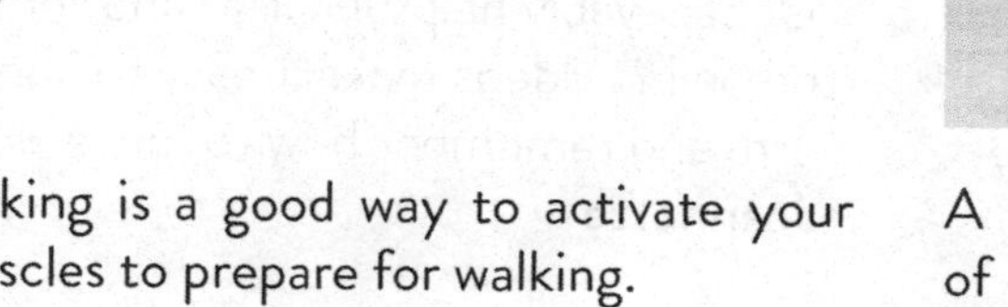

Tiptoe walking is a good way to activate your gluteal muscles to prepare for walking.

Dorsal Night Splint

The calf/soleus muscle complex in the lower leg crosses the knee joint and, when tight, contributes to knee pain. This tightness typically occurs because of sleeping habits that point the toes down, placing the ankle in a position of plantarflexion. This shortens the calf/soleus complex for 6–8 hours, wiping away any lengthening that occurs during the day.

Wear a dorsal splint at night to hold the ankle in a neutral position while sleeping, maintaining the length of the calf/soleus complex. This will reduce the forces acting on the knee joint.

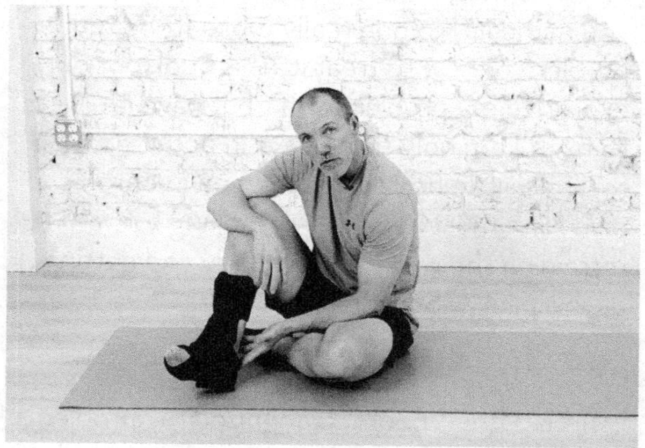

A dorsal night splint reduces the shortening of the calf/soleus complex that occurs while sleeping.

"The books in this series deserve WAY BEYOND a five-star rating. And to say the words 'Thank You' to Dr. Olderman seems like such an insignificant way of repaying him for his knowledge that is contained within these books!

"My experience has been great. Recovering from labrum surgery, I was concerned that I wouldn't be able to do some of the things I did before. However, I was back to 100% in about three months and was able to feel more confident in my shoulder than ever before." **-Jordan Norwood (Denver Broncos Superbowl Champion 2016)**

"Wow! I have gone to countless doctors, physical therapists, Pilates instructors, chiropractors, you name it. No one really understood my problem or how to treat it. This book not only explained my problem to a t but gave me ways to fix it. I am only three days in but already feeling a little better. I have been in chronic pain for almost 3 years. I'm looking forward to retraining the way I use my body and getting rid of this pain." **-Scott M**

"This is a great book. Recognized my problems in one of the client descriptions, followed the directions and within a month was pain-free ending over a year of bad hip pain." **-Amazon Customer**

"Do yourself a favor: get this book and do the exercises. You won't believe the difference it makes. I'm going to recommend it to everyone I know with any problems along this line. In fact, I've already recommended it to three people!" **-Amazon Customer**

"I think he is a truly kind person and a healer willing to go out of his way to help people and I have great respect for his knowledge! His books are clear and well-written." **-MJ**

"This book is an incredible resource. Olderman seems to thoroughly understand his subject and offer real solutions for common, yet complicated, complaints. The video links are an especially valuable reference tool." **-S Osborn**

"This one is a miracle worker. I was in terrible pain, and these exercises slowly helped heal. I still do most of them at least once a day. I highly recommend it." **-Sherl L**

"Unbelievably helpful. Clear and sensible, and the online videos make it easy to check your form and remember how to move well!" **-Jeannette**

BIOGRAPHIES

Rick Olderman, MSPT, is a sports and orthopedic physical therapist with more than 25 years' experience who specializes in helping people with chronic pain experience a pain-free life. Rick has created digital home programs to solve chronic, nagging or difficult pain. They can be found at **www.FixingYouMethod.com**.

Rick has created a practitioner training course for health and wellness professionals from coaches to surgeons that can be found at **www.HealPatientsFaster.com**.

Visit **www.RickOlderman.com** to see Rick's other products and free information.

Rick can be reached at **support@rickolderman.com.**

• • •

Rick's other books:

Solving the Pain Puzzle: Cases from 25 Years as a Physical Therapist, 2023
Fixing You: Back Pain 2nd ed., 2015
Fixing You: Hip & Knee Pain, 2011
Fixing You: Neck Pain & Headaches, 2009
Fixing You: Foot & Ankle Pain, 2012
Fixing You: Shoulder & Elbow Pain, 2010
Fixing You: Back Pain During Pregnancy, 2010

Bob Schrupp owned and ran a 50-person private practice firm that treated patients from 1990-2020. He also became a YouTube influencer in 2011, and he and Brad Heineck currently have 4.9 million subscribers. He has been married to the love of his life "Linda" since 1985. They have 3 children, Jamie, Sarah, and Matt. He lives with his wife in Winona, MN.

Made in the USA
Monee, IL
03 February 2024

52749986R00079